I0417059

The PMS Cure

Copyright © 2015 by Susan Richards, M.D.

All rights reserved. No part of this book may be reproduced or transmitted in any form or by any means, electronic or mechanical, including photocopying, recording, or by any information storage or retrieval system, without permission in writing from the Publisher.

Dr. Susan's Healthy Living
drsusanshealthyliving.com

Facebook.com/DrSusanRichards
drsusanshealthyliving@gmail.com
(650) 561-9978

Mention of specific companies or products in this book does not suggest endorsement by the author or publisher. Internet addresses and telephone numbers for resources provided in this book were accurate at the time it went to press.

ISBN 978-1511965880

Note

The information in this book is meant to complement the advice and guidance of your physician, not replace it. It is very important that any person who has medical problems be evaluated by a physician. If you are under the care of a physician, you should discuss any major changes in your regimen with him or her. Because this is a book and not a medical consultation, keep in mind that the information presented here may not apply in your particular case. In view of individual medical requirements, new research, and government regulations, it is the responsibility of the reader to validate health practices and treatments with a physician or health service.

Table of Contents

Introduction

Dear Friend,

I am so glad that you found my book, *The PMS Cure*. I wrote this book to share with you the most effective and fast acting all natural treatments for PMS that I have worked with as a medical doctor. My program has helped many thousands of my PMS patients who have experienced significant relief from their debilitating and uncomfortable PMS symptoms. I have developed my program not only through working with many patients but also having a thorough knowledge of the medical research in this field. In this book I have brought you the very best all natural, safe and effective PMS treatments!

Over the years I found that if I worked closely with my patients, together we could get better results than had ever seemed possible. Women who had been suffering from extreme premenstrual mood swings, irritability, bloating and uncontrollable food cravings were suddenly completely healed and full of energy and good spirit. Seeing people's lives and health improve so radically through my effective program has been a wonderful experience, and I am thrilled to share it with you.

Once my patients realized that the hormonal and chemical imbalances that trigger PMS symptoms often originated in unhealthy habits of diet, lack of exercise, and poor management of stress, they were very enthusiastic to make the positive lifestyle changes to become PMS free.

I provide my patients with many great resources to work with including, nutritional supplement guidelines, meal plans, recipes and stress reduction techniques. For my patients who want additional resources, I also share with them PMS relieving stretches, acupressure massage points and chiropractic techniques that also helped relieve their symptoms.

I wrote this book so that you could benefit from my all natural treatment program. I hope that you will find it as helpful and enjoy using it as much as my patients and I have.

Learning to Cure Myself

I first found out about PMS during my late teens when I began to suffer from uncomfortable symptoms each month. My menstrual periods, which had always been irregular, began to be preceded by bloating and weight gain of five to eight pounds. My hair became oilier and acne lesions and blemishes began to appear on my nose and cheeks.

During those years these was nothing for me to do except take aspirin. When I asked my mother for help she could only offer sympathy. She told me that I'd probably grow out of this problem as I got older. Instead, it got worse. My PMS continued all through my medical school training at Northwestern University. One week out of the month I was in too much pain to do my work easily.

I still remember the many afternoons when I had to leave the medical or pediatric ward because of my severe PMS symptoms and menstrual cramps. I went to the medical student on-call room and lay there in agony with severe nausea and cramps. My body swelled up so badly that I couldn't bear to bump against anything. The cysts in my breasts became large and tender.

My symptoms made me feel uncomfortable and different from the other students. My moods fluctuated terribly. Part of the month I would feel calm and relaxed like everyone else. But before my period I became more irritable and hard to deal with. I craved sugar and went on junk-food binges. Often I'd steal away and cry, not knowing how I was ever going to get through my training. I tried the accepted treatments, mild tranquilizers for my moods, antispasmodics for my cramps, and diuretics for my bloating. None of these medications worked particularly well.

Then, during my internship, everything changed. I was doing my specialty training and was expected to keep up with the current medical research in my field. One day an article came across my desk. It described work being done by doctors in Europe who were using high doses of vitamins to treat breast cysts. Excited by this, I spent the rest of the year hunting in the medical library for other information about treating menstrual disorders through nutrition.

I began to test a very simple program on myself, using high doses of vitamin B-complex and vitamin E. Somewhat to my surprise, this helped my sugar cravings, weight fluctuation, and bloating. Then I began to decrease the amount of sugar and caffeine in my diet. As a busy student, I had depended on "quick energy" foods like sweet rolls and coffee. Medical students were expected to help take care of a large ward of sick patients on little sleep. We needed all the energy we could get, but mealtimes allowed for little more than grabbing a few bites in the cafeteria.

I began to pay more attention to my diet, eating more whole grains and vegetables. I was amazed with the results: each month my menstrual symptoms were less severe. However, my mood swings and irritability persisted which I found very uncomfortable. I began to learn and practice a number of very relaxing and enjoyable stress reduction techniques. Since that time I finally became totally free of premenstrual symptoms and, thankfully, my menstrual periods were much more comfortable and easy to handle.

How a Self-Care Approach Can Work for You

PMS doesn't hit a victim at random like a thunderbolt. While we can be born with a predisposition towards PMS, the actual symptoms become much more severe through unhealthy lifestyle habits. Medication and therapeutic hormones can make you feel well very rapidly (as soon as thirty minutes after taking progesterone). But even women who have done very well on medical therapy often find that their symptoms return when they stop medication if they haven't made substantial changes in their lifestyle habits.

This is why self-care can be so important. We are leaving the era when patients went passively to doctors looking for "magic pills." The patients gave up control of their problem to the doctor. This was not good for the doctor or the patient. Health care should be a team effort. People should be informed as to the choices available and the physician should function as an educator as well as provide loving care and support. My PMS self-care program will help you to build a record of success and enhance your health and well-being. In addition, my lifestyle-based treatments like a therapeutic diet, nutritional supplements and stress reduction techniques do not have the harmful side effects that drugs do. They are safer and gentler methods and will greatly improve your general health and wellness as well as help to eliminate your PMS symptoms.

As I mentioned, I work with many self-help methods. A treatment plan that utilizes only one method like a prescription medication and purports to be the treatment for PMS will probably work for only a small percentage of women. I have found that my results are much better if I completely individualize each patient's treatment program.

For example, some women feel their best on a high carbohydrate, vegetarian emphasis diet while other women need a more meat-based high protein diet. Both of these types of diets can successfully help to eliminate PMS symptoms, as long as they are high in essential nutrients and eliminate foods that trigger these symptoms. As a result, I have included menus, meal plans and recipes in this book that provide you with both of these dietary options to fit your specific needs! I have also included stress reduction techniques, acupressure massage points, stretches, neurolymphatic and neurovascular points that you may find helpful in providing symptom relief.

You can read through the entire book first to familiarize yourself with the material or you can initially go to the treatment chapters that most appeal to you. Establish a regimen that works best for you and use it each month. This program is easy to follow and practical. It can be used by itself or in conjunction with a medical program. And best of all, it works. The feeling of wellness that can be yours with my PMS healing program will radiate out and touch your whole life. You will have more time and energy to enjoy your work, family, and other pleasures in life.

Love,

Dr. Susan

Part I:
The Problem

1

What Is Premenstrual Syndrome?

I want to start our program together by discussing the symptoms and risk factors of PMS. This is a very important part of your healing journey since so many varied symptoms have been linked to PMS. In fact, you may have symptoms that occur during the premenstrual time of the month and not have made the connection between how you feel and when these symptoms occur. Pinpointing your symptoms and risk factors will help you to better utilize the self-care treatments that I share with you later on in my book.

First, I would like you to understand that premenstrual syndrome is a very real health issue and it is not a myth. It takes its toll on the lives of millions of women. In fact, PMS is one of the most common female specific health problems affecting younger women. It is believed to impact between one third and one half of all American women between the ages of twenty and fifty — in other words, as many as twelve to twenty five million women.

Until I learned how to heal my own symptoms during my years of medical training, it took a terrible toll on my own life. If you are suffering from moderate to severe symptoms of PMS, it is probably having a major impact on your life, too.

The symptoms usually begin several days to as much as ten to fourteen days prior to the onset of the menstrual period and become progressively worse until the onset of menstruation or, for some women, several days after the onset. That means that millions of women go through half of each month of their adult life feeling sick. What this translates into in terms of lost productivity and quality of life is staggering.

The Symptoms

Let's look now at the symptoms of premenstrual syndrome. You will probably recognize many of your own symptoms in this list. The symptoms of PMS are numerous and affect practically every organ system of the body. More than 150 have been documented. Some of the most common ones are:

irritability	bloating	less frequent
anxiety	weight gain	urination
mood swings	constipation	asthma
depression	sugar craving	breast tenderness
hostility	cramps	breast swelling
migraine	acne	rhinitis
headache	boils	sore throat
dizziness	allergies	hoarseness
fainting	hives	joint pain and
tremulousness	cystitis	swelling
abdominal	urethritis	backache

Do you recognize yourself in this list? It is common for many of these symptoms to co-exist in the same women. My patients often report as many as ten or twelve symptoms. PMS seems to touch every aspect of their lives—from their relationships with family and friends, to their work productivity, to their ability to take pleasure in their own bodies.

There is a pervasive sense of "things are always falling apart" during the PMS period. Severely afflicted women are most vulnerable to extremes of behavior during this period. Women may experience an increased likelihood of accidents, alcohol abuse, suicide attempts, and, in rare cases, even crimes being committed by women when they are suffering from severe PMS.

While I don't often have patients who demonstrate such extreme aberrations, many of my women patients have described undergoing uncomfortable personality changes during the PMS time of the month. They will share with me that they are "irritable;' "grouchy" and "mean", that they yell at their children, pick fights with their spouses and snap at friends and co-workers prior to the onset of menstruation. They often spend the rest of the month repairing the emotional damage done to their relationships during this time. Often their children are bewildered and hurt, not understanding how mommy can suddenly turn so mean.

Often, my patients told me that they would turn to their physicians for help and would be offered only a tranquilizer or a psychiatric referral. Women would invest time and money in counseling that often didn't help. This would only add to their sense of failure and confusion about their medical problem.

Happily, my all-natural treatment program provided virtually every one of my patients with the relief that they were looking for. My program is based on self-care treatments that my patients could begin and start to notice almost instant relief form their PMS symptoms. I am thrilled that I can share my program with you, too.

The Factors That Increase Your Risk

Let's look now at the factors that place you at higher risk of developing PMS. Happily, modifying the risk factors that you can readily change, like beginning a PMS relief diet, taking therapeutic nutritional supplements and starting an exercise program can often have a dramatic impact on relieving your PMS symptoms! You are higher at risk of having PMS if:

- You have difficulty maintaining a stable weight.
- You do not exercise.
- You have a high stress diet with a significant intake of foods that trigger PMS symptoms.
- You do not take nutritional supplements.
- You are married.
- There is significant emotional stress in your life.
- You have had a pregnancy complicated by toxemia.
- You are over thirty. (The most severe symptoms occur in women in their thirties and forties.)
- You have suffered side effects from birth control pills. (Women who are unable to tolerate the pill seem to be more likely to get PMS.)
- You have children. (The more children, the more severe the symptoms.)

2

The Causes and Types of PMS

In this chapter, I want to describe the normal menstrual cycle and how it functions. This will give you a foundation to understand how your own f body works. This knowledge will make it much easier for you to understand the changes your body chemistry undergoes with PMS.

If you want to skip this information, you can go right on to the next section in which I discuss the different categories of PMS symptoms and the chemical and hormonal imbalances that may be contributing to each category.

The Purpose of Menstruation

Menstruation is the shedding of the lining of the uterus. This occurs each month with most women. The lining of the uterus (the endometrium) increases in thickness throughout the monthly cycle due to an increase in the blood supply and micronutrients. This thickening occurs to prepare a home for the fertilized egg during its nine months of growth and development within the mother's uterus. If pregnancy does not occur, then this lining is not needed. The uterus cleanses itself of the cells with the monthly bleeding. It then prepares the endometrium all over again the following month.

The Hormonal Feedback System

A cyclical pattern occurs because of the fluctuations in your hormonal levels. This is based on a feedback system in which the hormonal gland secretes a chemical (hormone), which enters the bloodstream and triggers a reaction in another gland often farther away. The hormone acts as a messenger, either giving another gland instructions to make its own hormone or triggering a chemical response in other parts of the body.

The hypothalamus, a glandular center located in the brain above the pituitary, is where hormones are produced that trigger the menstrual cycle. From this central location, it receives and sends nerve signals to many other parts of the brain. It regulates many functions, including hunger, thirst, sleep patterns, and all the endocrine functions, including menstruation. The hypothalamus is very sensitive to environmental stimuli such as emotional stress and physical illness.

Such stress can modify the signals that the hypothalamus passes on to the pituitary and from there on to the rest of the endocrine system. This can cause irregularities in the menstrual cycle. The hypothalamus communicates with the pituitary gland by releasing into the bloodstream messengers called FSH-RF (follicle-stimulating hormone-releasing factor) and LH-RF (luteinizing hormone-releasing factor). Their job is to tell the pituitary to make its own hormones.

From its position at the base of the brain, just below the hypothalamus, the pituitary produces the hormones needed to stimulate all the other glands of the body. Thus it has a very important regulating function. It stimulates the menstrual cycle by producing FSH (follicle-stimulating hormone) and LH (luteinizing hormone) as well as adrenocorticotropic hormone (ACTH) and the thyroid-stimulating hormone (TSH).

FSH and LH are released into the bloodstream with the ovaries as their destination. The ovaries are located in the woman's pelvic region and contain all the eggs that she will ever have. At birth each woman has between 100,000 and 400,000 eggs in an inactive form called follicles. They decrease progressively throughout her life until she reaches menopause, at which time most have been destroyed and the ovaries cease to function.

Each month, FSH and LH from the pituitary cause the follicles to ripen and one of them to grow into an egg. In doing so the follicle begins to produce the hormones estrogen and progesterone. Besides preparing the egg to be fertilized, these hormones also stimulate the lining of the uterus to prepare a proper home for the egg to grow. The estrogen and progesterone also control the obvious physical signs of femininity, such as breast development and growth of pubic hair. Sexual hormones in smaller amounts are also produced by the adrenal glands, which are located on top of the kidneys. As estrogen and progesterone circulate through the blood-stream they pass through the liver. The liver functions as a garbage disposal service. When high levels of hormones are no longer needed, it breaks them down and renders them chemically inactive so that they can be excreted from the body through your digestive tract, in your bowel movements. The kidney also excretes the chemically altered hormones into the urine and their passage through the body is complete.

The Monthly Cycle

On day 1, the first day of menstruation, estrogen and progesterone levels are extremely low. The hypothalamus reacts by releasing FSH-RF, which stimulates the pituitary to produce FSH. FSH stimulates the follicle cells of the ovary to begin increasing in size and producing estrogen. The increased amount of estrogen produced by these follicles stimulate the lining of the uterus to grow so that by mid-cycle it has increased three times in thickness and has a greatly increased blood supply.

One of the follicles, the Graafian follicle, surpasses the growth of the others and produces the egg for that month. At mid-cycle (day 14) and immediately prior to ovulation, estrogen levels reach their peak. This causes the pituitary to decrease the amount of FSH produced and increase the amount of LH. This triggers the release of the egg from the follicle and its extrusion from the ovary.

The egg is picked up by the Fallopian tube and stays there for twelve to thirty-six hours. It is during this time that the egg can be fertilized. Between mid-cycle and day 28, the LH causes the Graafian follicle left in the ovary to change into a corpus luteum, or yellow body. This yellow body produces high levels of estrogen and especially progesterone.

Adequate levels of progesterone are essential for maintaining a pregnancy. Progesterone causes the increase in basal body temperature seen at ovulation. It also causes a coiling of the blood vessels of the endometrium so that the lining becomes more compact.

The Types of PMS

The most common symptoms of which PMS patients complain can be broken down into four subgroups according to the classification system originally developed by Dr. Guy Abraham who was a clinical professor of obstetrics and gynecology at UCLA. Dr. Abraham published many research papers on the subject of PMS.

Type A (*for "anxiety"*): anxiety, irritability, mood swings, anger

Type C (*for "carbohydrates" or "cravings"*): sugar craving, fatigue, headaches

Type H (*for "hyperhydration"*): bloating, weight gain, breast swelling and tenderness

Type D (*for "depression"*): depression, "the blues," sadness, confusion, memory loss

I have added to these categories three other common subgroups that I have frequently seen with my patients.

Acne: pimples, oily skin and hair

Dysmenorrhea: cramps, low back pain, constipation, nausea, and vomiting. While dysmenorrhea is not a part of PMS, it is often seen with PMS symptoms.

Allergies: allergies, sinusitis, and asthma

Current medical research indicates that each symptom group is due to its own specific chemical and hormonal imbalances. Thus, PMS may be looked upon as at least seven different problem entities, often coexisting in the same woman.

Type A: Anxiety, Irritability, and Mood Swings. Type A is the most common subtype. Symptoms of anxiety, irritability, depression and mood swings often occurred in 80 to 90 percent of the women with this issue. The mood symptoms worsen in the days prior to the menstrual period and are relieved only with its onset.

One likely cause is an imbalance in the body's estrogen and progesterone levels. Both hormones increase during the second half of the menstrual cycle. When properly balanced, they promote normal function of the uterus, vagina, and breast. PMS mood symptoms occur if estrogens predominate, making women feel anxious. If progesterone predominates, women tend to feel depressed.

Physicians have been uncertain as to whether the emotional symptoms of PMS were due to an underlying psychiatric disorder. A research study reported in the *Annals of Medicine*, reported that women with PMS showed no more evidence of psychiatric or personality disorders than women without PMS, during their symptom-free periods, which suggests that PMS is more likely due to a chemical imbalance.

The balance between these hormones depends on two things: how much hormone is produced by the ovaries and how efficiently the hormone is broken down and disposed of by the liver and prepared for excretion by the kidney. Both emotional stress and nutritional habits can hamper how efficiently this system will run.

For example, stressful foods, such as excess fats, alcohol, and sugar, will overwork the liver, which must process them as well as the hormones. With vitamin B deficiency, which can be caused either by poor nutrition or by emotional stress, the liver does not have the raw material that it needs to carry out its metabolic tasks. In either case, the liver is unable to break down the hormones efficiently. This can increase the levels of estrogen or progesterone that continue to circulate in the blood without proper disposal.

Some researchers have linked the anxiety symptoms of PMS to insufficient levels of the neurotransmitter serotonin and the amino acid that produces it each day, tryptophan. When either serotonin or tryptophan levels are low, sleep problems, anxiety, irritability, and food cravings may occur.

Type C: Sugar Craving, Fatigue, and Headaches. Sixty to eighty percent of women with PMS notice an increased craving for refined carbohydrates, particularly sugar, chocolate, alcohol, white bread, pastries, white rice, and noodles. These women tend to eat large quantities of these foods before their periods. Their intention may be to eat a single cookie but women with these symptoms find that they end up eating the entire box of cookies. A few hours after indulging in refined carbohydrate foods many women complain of fatigue, headaches, shakiness, and dizziness.

Several mechanisms for the problem have been postulated. A woman's body is more responsive to insulin the week before her period starts. This tends to lower her blood sugar level because the insulin allows sugar to leave the bloodstream and enter the cells. With less circulating glucose, there is less sugar available for the brain, which uses up to twenty percent of the body's total energy supply.

Glucose is the major energy form, or fuel, of the body. The brain signals that more fuel is needed, and the body translates that signal into an increased craving for sweets. This craving is worse if she is under stress, because her brain then needs more fuel. It is also worse if her nutritional habits are poor and she lacks sufficient vitamin B, magnesium, and chromium in her diet. Without these nutrients, the body can't break down the sugar to use it for fuel.

In the premenstrual period many women crave chocolate. Chocolate is rich in phenylethylamine, which has an antidepressant effect (remember, depression is very common with PMS). Chocolate cravings may represent the body's need to find sources of nutrients that it is deficient in, but unfortunately, chocolate contains a number of ingredients that worsen PMS.

Type H: Bloating, Weight Gain, and Breast Tenderness. Women with Type H complain of abdominal bloating, breast tenderness, and weight gain. For many women, the subjective sensation of bloating is worse than the actual weight gain, which is seldom more than three pounds. With other women, the weight gain is more extreme, as much as five to ten pounds.

Some women may find that they need to have a second set of clothes or a larger size bra during the premenstrual period. They may find it difficult to take rings off and on their fingers or their legs may feel swollen. These women tend to retain excess fluid and salt due to excessive levels of estrogen in the body in comparison to the other female hormone, progesterone. As a result, you urinate less frequently.

In addition, imbalances in other hormones such as prolactin, the milk-release hormone secreted by the pituitary gland and the series-2 prostaglandin hormones, which are a primary cause of menstrual cramps, have also been linked to fluid retention symptoms. 60 to 70 percent of women with PMS experience these symptoms.

Type D: Depression, Confusion, Insomnia, and Memory Loss. Type D is the least common subgroup. Estrogen levels have been found to be low in women with Type D. Thus the depressant effects of high or normal progesterone are not counter-balanced by estrogen. Type D is potentially the most serious type of all because the women affected can be suicidal in severe cases. The depression also makes these women likely to become withdrawn, so that they are less likely to seek medical care.

Acne: Pimples and Oily Skin and Hair. Some women experience an increase in male hormones (androgens) from the adrenal gland in the time before their periods. This causes changes in the pH of the skin as well as an increase in the skin's oil secretion. Lesions may be found on the face, shoulders and back of susceptible women.

Acne can go through three stages. Blackheads are the mildest lesion. They occur when skin pores are blocked by oil. Most of the oil in the pore is white, but the oil that is exposed to the air on the skin surface turns black. Whiteheads are the second stage of acne. With this stage, the oil has no pore opening to the outside. Drainage cannot occur. Cysts form underneath the skin and become infected. This environment is perfect for the overgrowth of bacteria that cause the third stage, cystic acne. The cysts are hard and deep and can be painful to touch.

Dysmenorrhea: Cramps, Low Back Pain, Constipation, Nausea, and Vomiting. Cramps are often a young woman's introduction to discomfort surrounding the menstrual period. "Primary" dysmenorrhea often begins during the teenage years. It is due to spasm of the uterine muscles. Pain can also occur in the lower abdomen, lower back, and inner thighs. Dysmenorrhea was one of the commonest reasons that young girls were excused from classroom attendance when I was a teenager. Research has found that primary dysmenorrhea is due to an imbalance of chemicals produced by the uterus. These are called prostaglandins.

There are many subgroups of prostaglandins. In women without menstrual cramps the different prostaglandins are properly balanced. When there is an excess of series-2 prostaglandins (which causes cramping and pain) over series-1 prostaglandin (which has a muscle relaxant effect) cramps are the result.

Secondary dysmenorrhea may occur in women over thirty. It may be due in part to mechanical problems such as fibroid tumors. Pelvic inflammatory infections and endometriosis can cause scar tissue in the pelvic region. This can cause painful stretching with the onset of menses. Congestion caused by retention of fluid and sodium may also worsen pelvic pain.

Allergies: Allergies, Sinusitis and Asthma. PMS seems to affect immunity. A number of my patients have complained about the worsening of their allergy symptoms including nasal congestion, sinusitis, eye redness, tearing and irritation, increased sensitivity to allergens including certain foods and even the symptoms of asthma during the premenstrual period.

It is important to be aware that there is interplay between our immunity and the ebb and flow of our hormones and brain chemistry throughout the month. Not surprisingly, adrenal weakness can contribute to these immune related conditions. The adrenal glands, along with the ovaries, are the major site of female hormone production. In addition, the adrenals also produce natural anti-inflammatory substances that help to support your immunity and ability to suppress inflammation. Inflammation is a major characteristic of these allergic and respiratory conditions.

Part II:
Evaluating Your Symptoms

3

The PMS Workbook

Evaluating Your Symptoms

The self-evaluation questionnaires in this chapter will help you become more familiar with your own symptoms and the lifestyle factors that may be triggering your PMS symptoms. These questionnaires are very important to fill out since PMS is a diagnosis primarily based on your medical history of symptoms, rather than a diagnosis based on laboratory testing. There are no definitive lab tests for PMS! Thus, tracking your own symptoms and looking at your lifestyle habits is very important in resolving your PMS related issues.

If you take the time to fill out this calendar, you will find that this will make it easier for you to identify your symptoms, recognize your weak areas, and then follow the self-care treatment program from the chapters that follow.

First, fill out the monthly calendar of menstrual symptoms, starting with today. It is very helpful to make several copies of it before you start. The calendar will allow you to classify your symptoms and see whether they cluster around a particular type or types. This will make it easier for you to pick the specific treatments for your symptoms. Keep the monthly calendars to check your progress.

After you have filled out the calendar for today, turn to the evaluations that follow the calendar section. They will help you assess specific areas of your life to see which of your habit patterns are contributing to your PMS. When you've completed the evaluations, you will be ready to go on to Part III and begin your treatment program.

Monthly Calendar of Menstrual Symptoms

Grade your symptoms as you experience them each month

Date _____

Legend: ○ None   ✓ Mild   ◗ Moderate   ● Severe

DAY OF CYCLE	1	2	3	4	5	6	7	8	9	10	11	12	13	14	15	16	17	18	19	20	21	22	23	24	25	26	27	28	29	30	31
TYPE A																															
Nervous tension																															
Mood swings																															
Irritability																															
Anxiety																															
TYPE C																															
Headache																															
Craving for sweets																															
Increased appetite																															
Pounding heart																															
Fatigue																															
Tremulousness																															
TYPE D																															
Depression																															
Forgetfulness																															
Crying																															
Sleeplessness																															
TYPE H																															
Weight gain																															
Swelling of extremities																															
Breast tenderness																															
Abdominal Bloating																															
DYSMENORRHEA																															
Cramps (low abdominal)																															
Backache																															
General aches and pains																															
Nausea and vomiting																															
ACNE																															
Oily skin																															
Oily hair																															
Pimples																															

Eating Habits and PMS

Check off the number of times you eat the following foods:

Foods That Increase Symptoms

Foods	Never	1x a Month	1x a Week	>1x a Week
Coffee				
Cow's milk				
Cow's cheese				
Butter				
Chocolate				
Sugar				
Alcohol				
White bread				
White noodles				
White-based flour				
Pastries				
Added salt				
Bouillon				
Salad dressing				
Catsup				
Black tea				
Soft drinks				
Hot dogs				
Ham				
Bacon				
Beef				
Lamb				
Pork				
Salami				

Foods That Decrease Symptoms

Foods	Never	1x a Month	1x a Week	>1x a Week
Avocado				
Green Beans				
Beets				
Broccoli				
Brussels sprouts				
Cabbage				
Carrots				
Celery				
Collard greens				
Cucumbers				
Eggplant				
Garlic				
Horseradish				
Kale				
Legumes				
Lettuce				
Mustard greens				
Okra				
Onions				
Parsnips				
Peas				
Potatoes				
Radishes				
Rutabagas				
Spinach				
Squash				
Sweet potatoes				
Tomatoes				
Turnips				
Turnip greens				
Yams				
Brown rice				
Millet				
Barley				
Oatmeal				
Buckwheat				
Rye				
Raw flaxseeds				
Corn				

Raw sesame seeds				
Raw sunflower seeds				
Raw almonds				
Raw filberts				
Raw pecans				
Raw walnuts				
Raw pumpkin seeds				
Apples				
Bananas				
Berries				
Pears				
Seasonal fruits				
Corn oil				
Flax oil				
Olive oil				
Sesame oil				
Safflower oil				
Eggs				
Poultry				
Fish				

Key to Eating Habits and Your PMS. All the foods in the shaded area are high-stress foods that can worsen your symptoms of PMS. If you eat a significant number of these foods, or if you eat any of these foods frequently, your nutritional habits may be contributing significantly to your symptoms.

All the foods from avocado to fish are high-nutrient, low-stress foods that may help to relieve or prevent PMS symptoms and should be included frequently in your diet. If you are already eating many of these foods and few of the high-stress foods, chances are your nutritional habits are good, and nutrition may not be a significant factor in your PMS. Stress-reduction and the exercises and other body work methods may be more important to you.

Exercise Habits and PMS

Check off the number of times you do any of the following:

Exercise	Never	1x a Month	1x - 2x a Wk	>2x a Week
Fast walking				
Running				
Swimming				
Bicycling				
Tennis				
Aerobic activity				
Stretches				
Other exercise				

Key to Exercise Habits and PMS. Exercise is a good outlet for stress and can improve oxygenation and reduce pain. If your total number of exercise periods per week is less than three, you will probably be more prone to multiple PMS symptoms, and the chapters on various kinds of exercise for PMS will be important to you.

If you are exercising more than three times a week, keep doing your exercises; they are probably making your symptoms less severe. You may want to add specific corrective exercises to your present regime, choosing them to fit your individual symptoms from the treatment chart.

Stress and PMS

Check the places where tension most commonly localizes in your body:

o Shoulders

o Neck and Throat

o Grinding Teeth

o Lower Back

o Headache

o Eyestrain

o Arms

o Stomach Muscles

Key to What Stress Does to Your Body. This evaluation should help you to become aware of where you sequester stress in your body. Everyone has her own favorite area: tensions automatically accumulate there, like nuts in a squirrel's cheek. This accumulation increases your general level of fatigue and lowers your energy. Storing tension in the spine can worsen cramps; storing it in the neck can cause headaches.

Try to remain aware of the areas where you store tension. When you feel tension building up in them, begin deep breathing. Often this will release the tension immediately. If it does not, use one of the other methods given in the chapter on stress reduction.

Major Stress Evaluation

Value	Score	Life Events
100	_____	Death of spouse
73	_____	Divorce from spouse
65	_____	Separation from spouse
63	_____	Death of a close family member
53	_____	Personal injury or illness (serious)
50	_____	Embark on a new marriage
47	_____	Fired from your steady job
45	_____	Have a marriage reconciliation
45	_____	Enter into retirement from work
44	_____	Change in health of a family member
40	_____	Learn that you are pregnant
39	_____	Difficulties with your sexual abilities
39	_____	Gaining a new family member
39	_____	Have a readjustment (major) in business
38	_____	Have a radical change in finances
37	_____	Death of a close relative
36	_____	Change to a different line of work
35	_____	Increase in number of marital arguments
31	_____	Take on a loan or mortgage of more than $70,000
30	_____	Foreclosure of mortgage or loan
29	_____	Responsibilities change at work
29	_____	Son or daughter leaving home
29	_____	Irritating trouble with in-laws
28	_____	Recognition for outstanding achievements
26	_____	Spouse begins or stops work
26	_____	You begin or end schooling
25	_____	You undergo a change in living conditions
24	_____	You revise your personal habits
23	_____	You experience trouble with your boss
20	_____	Work hours or conditions are different
20	_____	You change your residence
20	_____	You change your school or major subject

19	_____	Alterations in your recreation are marked
19	_____	Church or club activities change
18	_____	Social activities change
17	_____	Take on a loan or mortgage of less than $70,000
16	_____	Your sleeping habits change
15	_____	The number of family get-togethers changes
15	_____	Eating habits are altered
13	_____	You go on vacation
12	_____	The year-end holidays occur
11	_____	You commit a minor violation of the law
	_____	TOTAL

This evaluation has been modified from the Life Change Index developed by Dr. Thomas Holmes and his co-workers at the University of Washington Medical School.

Key to Major Stress Evaluation. A score of over 300 points on this evaluation indicates major life stress and vulnerability to serious illness. If you scored over 300, do everything you can to be good to yourself. Eat well, exercise and learn the methods for managing stress given in the chapter on stress reduction.

If you scored between 200 and 299, you are also at some risk of illness and should follow the suggestions above.

If you scored below 200, you are believed to be at low risk of illness caused by stress. But since stresses too small to figure in this evaluation may also play a part in your PMS, and since it is impossible to predict or prevent the occurrence of certain major stresses, it would still be helpful for you to learn the methods outlined in the chapter on stress reduction.

Daily Stress Evaluation

Check each item that seems to apply to you.

Work

- **Pushing too hard.** Too much responsibility is heaped on you or you push yourself too hard. You worry about getting it all done and doing it well.

- **Understimulation.** Work is boring. The lack of stimulation makes you tired. You wish you were somewhere else.

- **Time pressure.** You worry about getting your work done on time. You always feel rushed.

- **Boss pressure.** Your boss demands too much. Your boss is too picky.

- **Uncomfortable physical plant.** Lights are too bright or too dim, noises are too loud. You are exposed to noxious fumes or chemicals. There is too much activity going on around you, making it difficult to concentrate.

Husband or Significant Other

- **Communication.** Not enough discussion of feelings. You both tend to hold in emotion. Too much negative emotion and drama. You are always upset and angry. Not enough peace and quiet.

- **Discrepancy in communication.** One person talks about feelings too much, the other person too little.

- **Affection.** You do not feel that you receive enough affection. There is not enough holding, touching, and loving in your relationship. You are made uncomfortable by your partner's demands.

- **Sexuality.** Not enough sexual intimacy. You feel deprived by your partner. There is a demand for too-frequent sexual relations by your partner. You feel pressured.

- **Children.** They make too much noise. They make too many demands on your time.

o **Organization.** Home is poorly organized. It always seems messy, chores are half-finished.

o **Time.** Too much to do, never enough time to get it all done.

o **Responsibility.** You need more help. Too many demands on your time and energy.

The Inner You

o **Too much anxiety.** You worry too much about every little thing. You constantly worry about what can go wrong.

o **Victimization.** Everyone is taking advantage of you or wants to hurt you.

o **Poor self-image.** You don't like yourself enough. You are always finding fault with yourself.

o **Too critical.** You are always finding fault with others.

o **Inability to relax.** You are always wound up. It is difficult for you to relax.

o **Not enough self-renewal.** You don't play enough or take enough time off to relax and have fun.

o **Insufficient sleep.** You don't get enough sleep and often feel tired.

Key to Daily Stress Evaluation. This evaluation is included to help you become aware of the minor daily stresses in your life. Although these stresses are not as significant individually as major life stresses and are more difficult to quantify scientifically, they can build up and add significantly to your PMS and other health problems. Becoming aware of them is the first step toward lessening their effects on your life. Methods for reducing them and helping your body to deal with them are given in the chapter on stress reduction.

Part III:
Finding the Solution

4

The Premenstrual Syndrome Healing Program

The self-care chapters of this book will be very helpful in providing you with the relief and healing that you are looking for. I am certain that these healing resources will be as beneficial for you as they have been for so many of my patients as well as myself.

In the chapters that follow, you'll find helpful self-care treatments. These include my dietary and nutritional supplements program, menus, meal plans and delicious recipes. I have included chapters on stress reduction, exercise, acupressure points, chiropractic treatment points and stretching programs. In doing the exercises or stretches, I recommend that you choose the exercises that are focused on your combination of symptoms.

There are two ways that you can work with the treatment chapters. You can either begin by going to the chapters that most appeal to you and work with those therapies, first. However, I do recommend that you start right away by reading the dietary and nutritional supplement chapters, no matter what other chapters you work with.

The PMS relief diet and the therapeutic nutritional supplement program are essential to successfully eliminate your PMS symptoms. You can also read straight through the rest of the book, get a general overview of the various approaches, and find those you are interested in trying. Establish the regimen that works for you and use it each month. Whichever way you choose to approach the treatment chapters, if you follow the program faithfully, you will begin to see great improvements in your symptoms very quickly— often within a month or two. My program will also support your general health and well-being. Many of my patients have been thrilled that they have also enjoyed more energy, vitality, clarity of mind and resistance to illness by following these recommendations.

5

The Women's Diet: Nutrition For a Life Free of PMS

It is impossible to overestimate the importance of good nutrition in controlling PMS. No medication can entirely overcome the effects of a poor diet. Many patients who consult with me are often eating unhealthy foods that trigger their PMS symptoms to such a degree that they are having difficulty functioning in their careers and personal relationships during the PMS time of the month.

Once they begin following my special Women's Diet, not only do my patients rapidly become free of their PMS symptoms, but they also have more energy and a greater sense of wellbeing than they have had in years. Often, they find that symptoms they had never associated with PMS, such as allergies, frequent colds, sinusitis and panic episodes have disappeared, too, with a healthier diet.

I call the diet the Women's Diet rather than the PMS diet because it is more than just the sum of our knowledge about what is bad and what is good for PMS. It is really the diet that every woman above the age of puberty should follow (with small adjustments for pregnancy and menopause) in order to be in the best possible health.

The list of foods that worsen PMS includes many unhealthy staples of the American diet that many women automatically turn to when they feel tired and want a quick boost of energy (or when they feel depressed and seek solace in food).

But the fact is that these unhealthy foods have almost all become important in our diet within the last hundred years. Many of them are truly addictive and have the importance they do in our diet because they cause cycles of binging and hunger. These include caffeinated beverages, sugar, alcohol, chocolate, salt and other less obvious foods, such as dairy products and wheat.

I have found in my clinical practice that many of my patients are able to eliminate these offending foods very quickly and make healthier substitutions in their diet. They are able to make these changes almost immediately or within one to two menstrual cycles. Other women make the transition more slowly and the process can take a number of months to eliminate the PMS symptom causing foods. But once you make this transition, they will exert much less attraction, particularly in comparison to the delicious and healthful new foods you will have added to your diet.

Fortunately, the list of foods that are good for PMS is also a long one. And once you learn the knack of preparing them you will enjoy their delicious flavors and benefit greatly from their wide range of healthy nutrients.

The women's diet is very exciting and delicious. I think that you will enjoy the many menus, meal plans and recipes that I share with you later on in this book. The dishes that I have included are delicious, easy to prepare and very beneficial for your health. Many of these meals can be prepared in less than fifteen to twenty minutes and require only a few ingredients.

There is also no reason to sacrifice the fun of entertaining. The foods in the women's diet are delicious and nutritious and they will also benefit your entire family!

In the guidelines that follow, I explain the physiology behind the women's diet in the terms of Western medicine. Interestingly, for women who are interested in Traditional Chinese Medicine (TCM), the same foods would be indicated in this health model, too.

TCM presents the world as a balance of opposing elements: yin, which covers all those body elements, health conditions and foods that are cool, passive, negative, sugar-containing, water-containing, and expansive; and yang, which describes those that are hot, active, positive, salt-containing, and contracting.

Yin foods include candies, soft drinks, white flour, and milk products. Yang foods include meat, salty and pickled foods. Neutral foods include selections such as whole grains, legumes, fish, vegetables, sea vegetables, and temperate climate fruits that are beneficial for PMS. To eat predominantly at either end of the spectrum is considered stressful to the body and likely to predispose to disease. Interestingly enough, extreme yin and extreme yang foods are identical to high-stress foods that may worsen PMS in the Western model.

Foods That Worsen PMS

The Women's Diet limits, first and foremost:

- Foods that are high in refined sugars, caffeine, alcohol, chocolate, salt, dairy products, wheat and saturated fats.
- Foods that are highly processed and full of food additives.

Avoid Caffeinated Beverages, including coffee, tea, and cola drinks. Caffeine can worsen irritability, breast tenderness, anxiety, mood swings, and depletes the body's stores of vitamin B, thus interfering with carbohydrate metabolism.

A study reported in the *American Journal of Public Health* questioned 216 college students about the severity of their PMS symptoms in relationship to their caffeine intake. Only 16% of the students who used no caffeine reported severe symptoms. In contrast, 60% who drank more than 4.5 cups of caffeinated beverages per day reported severe symptoms.

Substituting water-processed decaffeinated coffee is often the easiest substitute to start with for those women who like the flavor of coffee. Coffee substitutes that are grain-based, such as Postum and Cafix, are even better.

Ginger tea is a stimulant that can actually be therapeutic for women with fatigue, since it has a vitalizing and energetic effect. Green tea also has many health benefits including promoting weight loss. It contains very little caffeine and can be used by most women with PMS. The one exception is that some women with anxiety and panic attacks are sometimes very sensitive to any level of caffeine intake and can't even tolerate the small amount contained in green tea.

Avoid caffeinated soft drinks and instead try a glass of sparkling water with a slice of lemon or lime and a dash of bitters. This is a great festive drink to enjoy at home or even at social events and get-togethers.

Avoid Alcohol. It depletes the body's level of vitamin B and minerals, disrupts carbohydrate metabolism, and intensifies symptoms of Type C PMS. Alcohol is toxic to the liver and can disrupt the liver's ability to metabolize hormones, thus causing higher than normal estrogen.

Substitute Nonalcoholic Beverages. You may occasionally use light wine or beer in small amounts. They have a lower alcohol content than hard liquor, liqueurs, and regular wine. A nonalcoholic cocktail such as mineral water with a twist of lime or lemon or a dash of bitters is an even better substitute.

Avoid Sugar. It depletes the body's B-complex vitamins and minerals and intensifies sugar craving and the symptoms of Type C. A study in the *Journal of Reproductive Medicine* compared premenstrual health with dietary habits. The consumption of sugary foods such as juices, colas, chocolate, and alcoholic beverages were correlated with the most severe PMS symptoms.

Substitute Stevia, Xylitol, maple syrup, honey and other sugar substitutes. Stevia is an herbal sweetener that is calorie free. Thus, it is helpful if you are on a weight loss program or don't want the extra calories found in other sweeteners such as sugar or honey. Because stevia contains no calories from sugar, it does not create imbalances in the blood sugar level. This is very beneficial if you suffer from hypoglycemia or diabetes.

Xylitol is a wonderful sweetener that is derived from woody fibrous plant material. It gives a delicious flavor to baked goods, desserts and beverages without the health problems related to table sugar like diabetes, candida infections, overweight and tooth decay. Even better, xylitol is as sweet as sugar but has only two thirds the calories.

Xylitol is absorbed more slowly than sugar so is helpful for diabetes, has antibacterial and antifungal properties and helps promote healthy teeth and gums. It is also found naturally in guavas, pears, blackberries, raspberries, aloe vera, eggplant, peas, green beans and corn.

Honey is two and a half times as sweet as sugar. Maple syrup is also sweeter and more concentrated than sugar. Substitute these in smaller amounts. Apple sauce and bananas can also be used as a substitute in baking.

Avoid Dairy Products, including milk, cheese, butter, cream, ice cream, and yogurt. Dairy interferes with the absorption of magnesium, a mineral that can decrease cramps, help glucose metabolism, and stabilize mood swings. Their high sodium content can worsen fluid retention and bloating, and their high saturated fat content decreases the liver's efficiency in metabolizing female hormones.

In addition, the fat contained in dairy products is the raw material that the body uses to make series-2 prostaglandin hormones, which have been linked to menstrual cramps, bloating, and mood swings. Elimination of even nonfat milk and yogurt can decrease symptoms like fatigue and abdominal bloating.

Substitute rice, almond, coconut, soy, flaxseed, hemp and sunflower seed milk. These are good sources of calcium and can be used for drinking, eating with cereal, or baking. Nondairy milks can also be substituted for milk or cream as a thickener for sauces.

As a substitute for butter, flax oil is golden, buttery, and delicious. It is perishable and must be kept sealed and refrigerated. It must not be used for cooking and should not be heated. Prepare your rice, baked potatoes, steamed vegetables and garlic bread first. Just before serving, mix in the flax oil.

Avoid Wheat and Gluten-Containing Grains. While consuming whole grains has many health benefits, some women with PMS and other estrogen dominant conditions like fibroid tumors may find that they are allergic to or intolerant of wheat. Most women are surprised by this discovery, since wheat is one of the staples of our culture and is eaten by most people at almost every meal. However, wheat contains a protein called gluten, which is highly allergenic and difficult for the body to break down, absorb, and assimilate. Women with a wheat intolerance are prone to fatigue, depression, sinusitis, allergies, bloating, intestinal gas, and bowel changes.

In my clinical experience, when women are nutritionally sensitive, wheat consumption can often worsen emotional symptoms and lower energy levels. I have observed how wheat (along with other foods) can trigger emotional symptoms, bloating and fatigue in PMS patients, especially during the week or two before the onset of menses.

Many menopausal women also tolerate wheat poorly because their digestive tracts are beginning to show the wear and tear of aging and don't produce enough enzymes to break down wheat easily.

Women with allergies often find that wheat intensifies nasal and sinus congestion, as well as fatigue. I also find that women with poor resistance and a tendency toward infections may need to eliminate wheat from their diets to boost their immune systems. Since wheat is leavened with yeast, it should also be avoided by women with candida.

Substitute gluten-free grains. If you suffer from any of these conditions, along with PMS, you should probably eliminate wheat from your diet and use the many gluten-free breads, breakfast cereals, bagels, English muffins, cookies, pasta and other flour based foods that are readily available in health food stores and many supermarkets.

Oats and rye, which also contain gluten, should be eliminated along with wheat if your symptoms are moderate to severe. Gluten-free oats, however, are available in health food stores and some supermarkets.

I have found over the years that the least stressful grains for women with PMS symptoms are grains like brown rice, millet, quinoa, wild rice, amaranth and buckwheat. For example, buckwheat is not commonly eaten in our culture, so most women never develop an intolerance to it. Also, it is not in the same plant family as wheat and other grains. Buckwheat is actually the fruitlike structure of the plant rather than a grass. Other infrequently used grains such as wild rice, quinoa, and amaranth should be tried as well. These are available in health food stores in pastas and cereals.

Avoid Chocolate. It worsens mood swings, intensifies sugar craving, causes weight gain, and increases demand for the B-complex vitamins. It also causes breast tenderness.

Substitute unsweetened carob. It tastes like chocolate but is far more nutritious (although it is high in calories and fat and should be eaten in small amounts). It is a member of the legume family and is high in calcium. It can be purchased in chunk or chip form as a substitute for chocolate candy or as a powder to be used in baking or drinks. The magnesium that chocolate provides can be found in many other foods which I have included in a chart later on in this book.

Substitutes for Common High-Stress Ingredients

¾ cup sugar	¾ cup xylitol
	1/2 cup honey
	1/4 cup molasses
	1/2 cup maple syrup
	1/2 ounce barley malt
	1 cup apple butter
	2 cups apple juice
1 cup milk	1 cup soy, rice, nut, or grain milk
1 tablespoon butter	1 tablespoon flax oil (must be used raw and unheated)
½ teaspoon salt	1 tablespoon miso
	1/2 teaspoon potassium chloride salt substitute
	1/2 teaspoon Mrs. Dash, Spike
	1/2 teaspoon herbs (basil, tarragon, oregano, etc.)
1 ½ cups cocoa	1 cup powdered carob
1 square chocolate	3/4 tablespoon powdered carob
1 tablespoon coffee	1 tablespoon decaffeinated coffee
	1 tablespoon Postum, Cafix, or other grain-based coffee substitute
4 ounces wine	4 ounces light wine
8 ounces beer	8 ounces near beer
1 cup white flour	1 cup barley flour (pie crust)
	1 cup rice flour (cookies, cakes, breads)

Foods That Help PMS

An article in *American Family Physician*, found that a well-balanced diet low in saturated fats, but with adequate amounts of complex carbohydrates, protein, and fiber, and with a minimum intake of caffeine, alcohol, and salt is most beneficial for the relief of PMS symptoms.

The Women's Diet emphasizes the use of whole fresh foods. It is a return to the diet to which our bodies adapted over thousands of years. It emphasizes:

Foods Made from Whole Grains

Whole Grains. Whole grains (including corn, barley, gluten-free oats, rye, millet, buckwheat and brown rice) are complex carbohydrates, capable of stabilizing your blood sugar and helping tremendously to eliminate premenstrual sugar craving. They contain excellent sources of protein, fiber, vitamins B and E, and various minerals.

They can be prepared in a variety of ways. I generally tell women with PMS to avoid wheat as I have found that wheat increases bloating, weight gain, and gas. This may be due to the gluten content of wheat, which is difficult to digest and to which many people are highly allergic. Whole grains can be found at health food stores and most local supermarkets.

Whole-Grain Cereals. Whole-grain cereals, either hot or cold, will help your PMS. Some local supermarkets offer whole-grain cereals and gluten-free grains, while health food stores offer a larger choice of cereals and whole grain products. Puffed millet, puffed corn, and puffed rice are all available as cold breakfast cereals. Unsweetened granolas, gluten-free oats, cream of rye and buckwheat groats are also good.

Whole-grain Bread. Take advantage of the many different whole-grain breads that are available at supermarkets and health food stores today — rice, sesame-millet, gluten-free oatmeal, quinoa, soy-potato, rye, and lima bean bread, among others. Choose brands without added sugar.

Crackers. Crackers can be used for snacks or open-faced sandwiches. Brown rice cakes are a particularly good snack. Spread with nut butters or fruit preserves, they help stabilize the blood sugar level in women.

Pancakes and Waffles. Pancakes and waffles can be made with gluten-free oats, corn, buckwheat, or rice flour. Concentrated forms of sweeteners such as maple syrup, honey, and applesauce can be used in small amounts.

Pasta. When the word pasta is mentioned, most women think of refined wheat noodles and spaghetti. As I mentioned earlier, wheat worsens PMS bloating, weight gain, and gas for many women. It is very easy now, however, to find pasta made from other gluten-free grains such as buckwheat, quinoa, rice, corn, and soy. Whole grain pasta is also made with several delicately flavored vegetables, including artichokes and spinach.

Legumes

Lentils, kidney beans, pinto beans, mung beans, garbanzo beans, adzuki beans, green peas, are also equally beneficial for the relief of PMS symptoms. Because of their high complex carbohydrate and protein content, they help to regulate blood sugar levels thereby stabilizing mood swings, anxiety, and energy levels. When eaten with grains they form a complete protein comparable to that in eggs or meat. Legumes are also a great source of dietary fiber, and essential nutrients like potassium, calcium, iron, zinc and folic acid.

Tofu and other soybean-based foods are the base of many Asian diets. However, soybean-based foods are increasingly used in Western diets and are now readily available at most supermarkets.

Soybeans are an excellent food for women with PMS since they are an excellent source of plant estrogens. Plant estrogens actually help to relieve PMS symptoms by competing with your own level of estrogen when it is too high. Thus, the use of soy products helps to normalize your estrogen levels, thereby reducing PMS symptoms. In addition, soy beans are an excellent source of essential fatty acids, vegetable protein, calcium, potassium, vitamin C, and other important nutrients.

High protein soy-based products like tofu and tempeh are used by many women in stir-fry, casseroles, and pasta dishes as meat substitutes. In addition, many dairy substitute products are now available made from soy. These healthful and easy-to-digest products include soy milk, soy yogurt, soy cheese, soy sour cream, and even soy-based ice cream.

Still, soy is not for everyone. Some women don't like the taste of soy foods and other women have difficulty digesting it. It is one option among many that you can choose from to help relieve menopause symptoms.

If you are allergic to soy, then obviously you need to avoid consuming it entirely. If you find that soy foods cause digestive upset such as gas, bloating, or intestinal discomfort, I suggest taking a high-potency digestive enzyme such as bromelain or papain whenever you consume soy foods, or simply opt for supplemental soy isoflavones capsules.

Seeds and Nuts

Seeds and nuts are excellent sources of protein. They should be raw and unsalted. Never eat nuts and seeds that have been roasted, salted or coated with sugar as they will only worsen your symptoms. They are very high in calories so quantities consumed should be moderate if premenstrual weight gain is a problem for you. If you have acne, eat only very small amounts.

Vegetables

Leafy green vegetables such as kale, collard, and mustard greens, root vegetables such as rutabagas, carrots, turnips, and parsnips, and the cruciferous green vegetables such as broccoli and Brussels sprouts, are high in vitamin A, magnesium, calcium, and other nutrients that relieve PMS symptoms.

Red, orange, and yellow vegetables such as carrots, peppers, sweet potatoes, and squash, are high in complex carbohydrates and fiber, also help to reduce PMS-related hypoglycemia and mood swings. Their high vitamin A content helps to regulate heavy menstrual bleeding and premenstrual acne.

Fruits

The best fruits for PMS are those that are seasonal and grown in temperate climates such as apples and pears. They tend to be higher in fiber and lower in sugar content. Fruits grown in the hot tropical sun tend to be much sweeter, which can worsen fluid retention and sugar craving in susceptible women. If included as a part of your diet, tropical fruits are best eaten in the summer and as a topping for non dairy yogurt and gluten-free pancakes, waffles, muffins and other baked goods.

Poultry and Fish

I generally recommend eating red meat in moderation. If you want to eat meat, I recommend that you eat poultry, eggs or fish that are high in omega-3 fatty acids. Particularly good are omega -3 fatty acid containing fish like salmon, tuna, trout, halibut and mackerel. These fatty acids are converted within the body to the beneficial series-3 prostaglandins which help to reduce menstrual cramps. Fish should be eaten no more than once or twice a week due to the high mercury content in most fish.

I have found that fish oil capsules, when used as a nutritional supplement, are very helpful for my patients especially when you are eating a lot of foods like poultry, eggs and vegetarian diets that lack omega-3 fatty acids. Vegetarians can also obtain the omega-3 fatty acids, EPA and DHA, usually found in fish, from algae source supplements. Also, good meat options are free-range poultry, organic lean red meat, and game meat. Fatty cuts of red meats like beef, pork, and lamb contain the saturated fats that the body uses to produce the series-2 prostaglandins — the hormone-like chemicals that trigger muscle contraction and constriction in blood vessels, thereby worsening cramps.

I recommend that you increase your intake of grains, beans, and raw seeds and nuts, which contain protein as well as many other important nutrients, instead of using meat as your only or primary source of protein. For many years I have recommended to my patients that they use meat more as a garnish and a flavoring for casseroles, stir-fries, and soups.

I also recommend that you buy meat from organic, free-range, grass-fed sources; this meat has undergone less exposure to pesticides, antibiotics, and hormones. If you find meat difficult to digest, you may be deficient in hydrochloric acid, a digestive enzyme normally found in the stomach. Try taking a small amount of hydrochloric acid with every meat-containing meal to see if your digestion improves.

Oils

Preferred oils include sesame oil, olive oil, walnut oil, macadamia nut oil, corn oil, and safflower oil. Unlike animal fats, they are unsaturated. These are all monounsaturated and polyunsaturated oils. Cold-pressed oils tend to be fresher and purer. Flax oil is a great oil for using as a butter substitute but cannot but used for cooking because of its heat sensitivity. Food must be cooked first and then flax oil added before serving.

Healthy Food Shopping List

Vegetables

Beets	Eggplant	Radicchio
Bok choy	Garlic	Radishes
Broccoli	Green beans	Rutabagas
Brussels sprouts	Horseradish	Sauerkraut
Cabbage	Kale	Spinach
Carrots	Lettuce	Squash
Cauliflower	Mustard greens	Sweet potatoes
Celery	Okra	Tomatoes
Chard	Onions	Turnips
Cilantro	Parsley	Turnip greens
Collard	Parsnips	Watercress
Cucumbers	Peas (all varieties)	Yams
Dandelion greens	Potatoes	

Legumes
Adzuki
Black
Black-eyed peas
Cannellini
Fava
Garbanzo
Kidney
Lentils
Navy
Red
Soy: tofu, tempeh
Turtle beans

Whole Grains
Amaranth
Barley
Brown rice
Buckwheat
Corn
Millet
Oatmeal
Quinoa

Seeds and Nuts
Almonds
Cashews
Filberts
Flaxseeds
Macadamia
Pecan
Pumpkin seeds
Sesame seeds
Sunflower seeds
Walnuts

Healthy Food Shopping List (continued)

Fruits
Acai berries
Apples
Avocado
Bananas
Berries
Blueberries
Raspberries
Strawberries
Coconuts
Goji berries
Kiwi
Noni
Olives
Pomegranates
Pears
Seasonal fruits

Sweeteners
Brown rice syrup
Honey
Maple syrup
Molasses
Stevia
Xylitol

Beverages
Coconut water
Grain-based coffee
substitute
Herbal tea
Green tea
Water

Meats
Fish
Free-range poultry
Game meat
Organic lean red meat
Seafood (in
moderation)

Oils
Flax
Macadamia
Olive
Safflower
Sesame
Walnut

Foods from Other Cultures
Gomasio
Jicama
Miso
Seaweed (like kelp,
dulse, nori, wakane)
Tamari soy sauce
Umeboshi plums

Dairy Substitutes
Hemp milk
Nut milk
Rice milk
Soy milk
Soy, coconut, almond,
rice or hemp cheeses,
cream cheese, yogurt,
and frozen desserts
*Avoid all soy products
containing
hydrogenated oil.

Herbs & Spices
Basil
Black pepper
Cayenne pepper
Chamomile
Chili pepper, dried
Cilantro
Cinnamon, ground
Cloves
Coriander
Cumin
Dill
Ginger
Licorice
Mustard seeds
Oregano
Peppermint
Poppy
Rosemary
Sage
Tarragon
Thyme
Turmeric

6

Principles of the Women's Diet

Your Diet Should Provide the Greatest Possible Variety

Rotate your foods. This minimizes symptoms of food allergy, which can be worse before your period. It also guarantees that you will be taking in a larger range of nutrients. Many women fall into the rut of eating the same foods day after day. They will go to the same shelves of the supermarket out of habit and convenience.

There is safety in familiarity, sticking with a tried formula even if it adversely affects your health in the long run. Also, it takes time to learn new cooking methods. I have provided some very simple guidelines and shortcuts for food preparation that should help you get past the initial fear of trying a greater variety of foods.

Foods Should Be Simple and Easy to Prepare

Women today live very complex lives. Many have the responsibility of running households and holding full-time jobs. This leaves little time for meal-planning and cooking. It is no wonder so many women turn to convenience foods.

Fortunately, nutritious foods can be just as convenient as less nutritious foods. Over the years, my patients and I have worked out many shortcuts for preparing high-quality food. Many of them have used these shortcuts to great advantage, and can prepare a complete meal in fifteen to twenty minutes.

Nutritional Changes Should Be Fun

The suggestions in this book offer a chance to taste new types of food and try out new recipes. Approach tasting new foods as you would go to a new restaurant -- with a sense of excitement. Many people consider dietary changes a punishment and think that once their symptoms of PMS are better, they can go back to their old eating habits. But it is these habits that caused PMS in the first place, and they are something to be left behind.

To maximize your enjoyment of your new diet, emphasize the aesthetics of dining. A tablecloth, candles and attractive serving dishes can dress up even simple fare. Highlight the color and texture of each food by using side dishes for serving. Try to serve foods with complementary colors. You will be widening your choice of nutrients as well as increasing the eye appeal. (For example, red and yellow vegetables are high in vitamin A, while green vegetables are higher in vitamin C.) This attention to dining aesthetics will increase your emotional gratification and sense of well-being.

Meals Can Still Be Family Affairs

Eating to relieve PMS doesn't mean that you have to sit in a corner and eat by yourself. The nutritional suggestions made in this book can be used with benefit by all members of the family and friends. Most of my patients find that their families enjoy sharing the new foods, as well as feeling healthier.

Nearly all the dishes can be easily adapted to everyone's taste. If your children insist that life is empty without cheese or hamburger, add extra cheese and hamburger to one side of a casserole. Or prepare your side of a dish without the rich gravy that the rest of your family likes, or add more vegetables.

Chew Your Food Thoroughly

This is particularly important during the healing phase of PMS when you are trying to relieve the body of all significant stress. The first stage of digestion occurs in the mouth. Slow, thorough eating allows the food to be broken down before it reaches the stomach. Eating fast puts a strain in your digestive system. It will also cause you to eat more because you do not feel satiated until twenty minutes after you start eating. This can be a particular problem if weight gain or bloating is among your symptoms.

Eating high-stress foods like beef, dairy products, and sugary products can cause fatigue or a sensation of heaviness. The tiredness that so many women with PMS complain about can be exacerbated by these foods because so much energy is involved in the digestive process.

Eat Heavier Meals Early in the Day, Lighter Meals in the Evening

Digesting food while you are asleep puts a large metabolic load on your entire system. The night is the time when your body repairs itself. It is unhealthy during this rest period to ask your body to continue to work.

Changes Can Be Made Slowly

I have found in my medical practice that it takes anywhere from a month to two years to change one's dietary habits so that these changes feel comfortable and pleasurable (not just healthy). It is unrealistic to expect that you will throw away every high-stress food in your cupboard because you have PMS.

Look back at the list of foods that worsen PMS. Pick one or two foods from this list that you would be willing to give up immediately. Then look at the list of foods to substitute. For example, if you drink six cups of coffee a day and start your morning with orange juice, you might decide to switch to a coffee substitute like Postum and substitute a small piece of apple for the orange juice.

You may not want to make any other changes until a month later. When you are comfortable with these changes, go back to your list of foods to limit. Perhaps now you are ready to cut down on your intake of dairy products. Perhaps you could eliminate the slice of cheese from your sandwich at lunch. Instead of yogurt, you might take a bowl of soup.

Every few weeks go back to the list of foods to limit and foods to emphasize. Pick a few more foods to eliminate and a few more foods to add to your diet. Remember that even modest dietary changes can bring significant relief of your PMS. On the other hand, some people find it easier to change their diets by giving up foods abruptly, and that is fine too. The important thing is to find the way that will work for you.

7

More on Food Substitutions for PMS

While I discussed foods that worsen PMS and their substitutes in chapter 5, in this chapter I provide you with more detailed and very helpful information about the negative effects that these foods have on your PMS symptoms. You can read this chapter if you are interested in knowing more information about these high stress foods.

This information is based on extensive work with women who suffered from fatigue, depression, allergies, frequent colds and flus and other health issues and noted significant relief of their symptoms when following this program. It is also based on the medical research in this field.

Foods to Avoid

It is important to eliminate all foods that intensify your PMS symptoms. These include foods that are toxic and stressful to the body when used in excess, and that may trigger PMS symptoms in susceptible women when used even in small amounts. In my experience with patients suffering from moderate to severe PMS, all of these foods should be entirely eliminated or at least sharply curtailed to small amounts, used on an occasional basis as a treat.

Some women may find that they need to eliminate PMS-causing foods gradually because of their emotional or physical attachments to the food. When there are strong emotional attachments, the elimination process itself can cause stress; thus, it should be done gently. Many other women find that the "cold turkey" approach works best, and they appreciate the rapid relief from PMS symptoms that simply eliminating a stressful food brings. I will mention any pitfalls of such an approach when discussing the specific foods in this section.

Sugar

Glucose, a simple form of sugar, is the food that provides the body with its main source of energy. Without a steady supply of glucose, we could not produce the hundreds of thousands of chemical reactions our bodies need to perform daily functions. The brain is one of the primary users of glucose, requiring 20 percent of the total available glucose to function optimally.

However, the form in which you take this important food into your body can affect your mood in a profound manner. The ideal approach is to eat lots of complex carbohydrates such as whole grains, potatoes, fruit, and vegetables. The sugar in these foods digests slowly and is released into the blood circulation very gradually. Thus, the amount of sugar released from these foods does not overwhelm the body's ability to handle it.

Unfortunately, many Americans obtain their sugar intake through the excessive use of simple sugar—the refined white or brown sugar that is the primary ingredient of most cookies, candies, cakes, pies, soft drinks, ice cream, and other sweet foods. In addition, pasta and bread made from white flour, which has all the bran, essential fatty acids, and nutrients removed, act as simple sugars; unfortunately, these make up a significant part of the diet of many women in Western societies.

Many convenience foods, including salad dressing, ketchup, and relish, also contain high levels of both sugar and salt. With sugar so prevalent in many foods, sugar addiction is common in our society among people of all ages. Many people use sweet foods as a way to deal with their frustrations and other upsets. As a result, most Americans consume too much sugar—the average American eats 120 pounds per year.

This excessive level of sugar intake can be a major trigger of PMS food cravings, especially for carbohydrates. Here is what happens: Unlike complex carbohydrates, foods based on sugar and white flour break down quickly in the digestive tract. Glucose is released rapidly into the blood circulation and from there is absorbed by the cells of the body to satisfy their energy needs. To handle this overload, the pancreas must release large amounts of insulin, a chemical that helps move the glucose from the blood circulation into the cells.

Often the pancreas tends to overshoot the amount of insulin needed. As a result, the blood sugar level goes from too high to too low, resulting in the roller coaster effect typically seen in hypoglycemia or PMS. You may initially feel "high" after eating sugar, and then experience a rapid crash and a dip in your energy level. (Excessive amounts of stress also use up glucose rapidly and can cause similar symptoms.)

When your blood sugar level falls too low, you begin to feel anxious, jittery, spacey, and confused because your brain is deprived of its necessary fuel. To remedy this situation, the adrenal glands release cortisol and other hormones that cause your liver to release stored sugar so that your blood sugar can return to normal levels. Though the adrenal hormones boost the blood sugar level, they unfortunately increase arousal symptoms and anxiety too. Thus, both the initial glucose deprivation in the brain and the adrenal's response to restore the glucose levels can intensify symptoms of anxiety and panic in susceptible women in PMS.

Excessive use of sugar has further detrimental effects. Like caffeine, sugar depletes the body's B-complex vitamins and minerals, thereby increasing nervous tension, anxiety, and irritability. Too much sugar also intensifies fatigue by narrowing the diameter of the blood vessels and putting stress on the nervous system. Candida feeds on sugar, so overindulging in this high-stress food worsens chronic candida infections.

Many women with chronic candida complain of emotional symptoms like depression and nervous tension. Furthermore, sugar (as well as caffeine, alcohol, flavor enhancers, and white flour) appears to be an important trigger for the binge eating often seen with anxiety and PMS.

In fact, research studies have shown that when women switch from a diet high in sugar to a lower sugar, high-nutrient diet, food addictive behavior tends to cease. After making the switch from a high-sugar-intake diet, women tend to lose or maintain weight more easily and to successfully maintain relief from the pattern of craving and binging (for up to two years, in one study).

In summary, sugar stresses many bodily systems, worsens your health, and intensifies anxiety, nervous tension, and fatigue. Try to satisfy your sweet tooth instead with healthier foods. Consider fruit or grain-based desserts, like oatmeal cookies sweetened with fruit or honey. You will find that small amounts of these foods can satisfy your cravings. Instead of disrupting your mood and energy level, they actually have a healthful and balancing effect. Xylitol is a healthy sugar substitute that is actually beneficial for the teeth and gums. Xylitol can be used as a very good sugar substitute in recipes. Other sugar substitutes like stevia, rice bran syrup, maple syrup and molasses can also be used in small amounts.

Caffeine

Coffee, black tea, soft drinks, and chocolate all contain caffeine. Many women with PMS and high levels of stress mistakenly use caffeine as a pick-me-up to help them get through the day's tasks. Unfortunately, caffeine can trigger and aggravate anxiety and panic episodes in women with PMS.

Caffeine used in excess (more than four or five cups per day) can dramatically increase anxiety, irritability, and mood swings in general. Even small amounts can make susceptible women jittery. After the initial pick-up, women with anxiety coexisting with excessive stress find that caffeine intake makes them more tired than before.

Caffeine triggers anxiety and panic symptoms in women with PMS because it directly stimulates several arousal mechanisms in the body. It increases the brain's level of norepinephrine, a neurotransmitter that increases alertness. However, it also triggers sympathetic nervous system activity, which causes the fight-or-flight physiological responses in the body, such as increased pulse, breathing rate, and muscle tension. Thus, caffeine intake triggers the physiological responses typical of anxiety states. Also, caffeine stimulates the release of stress hormones from the adrenal glands, further intensifying symptoms of nervousness and jitteriness.

Caffeine depletes the body's stores of B-complex vitamins and essential minerals, such as potassium, which are important in the chemical reactions that convert food to usable energy. Deficiency of these nutrients increases anxiety, mood swings, and fatigue in women with PMS. Depletion of B-complex vitamins also interferes with carbohydrate metabolism and healthy liver function, which help to regulate the blood sugar as well as estrogen levels. An imbalance in estrogen and progesterone can increase anxiety and mood swings in women with symptoms of PMS.

If you suffer from moderate to severe anxiety symptoms due to PMS, I recommend that you reduce your caffeine consumption to one cup of coffee per day and try to eliminate cola drinks, caffeine-containing tea, and chocolate. Some women may find that going "cold turkey" with coffee and eliminating it abruptly causes unpleasant withdrawal symptoms such as headaches, depression, and fatigue. In these cases, it is better to cut down coffee intake gradually, decreasing the amounts slowly over a period of one month to several months, substituting first decaffeinated coffee and finally herbal teas. Many herbal teas, like chamomile and peppermint, even have a relaxant effect on the body, thereby helping to reduce anxiety.

Caffeine Content of Beverages and Foods
(listed in order of caffeine content)

	Caffeine per Serving
Coffee (per cup)	
Drip (average)	146 mg
Percolated (average)	110 mg
Coffee—instant (per cup)	
Folgers	97.5 mg
Maxwell House	94 mg
Nescafe	81 mg
Decaffeinated Coffee (per cup)	
Taster's Choice	3.5 mg
Tea (per cup)	
Tetley	63.5 mg
Lipton	52 mg
Constant Comment	29 mg
Green Tea	24-40 mg
Soft Drinks (per 12 oz. can)	
Mountain Dew	55 mg
Diet Dr. Pepper	54 mg
Coke Classic	46 mg
Diet Coke	46 mg
Pepsi	38.4 mg
Diet Pepsi	36 mg
Hot Chocolate Drinks (per cup)	
Cocoa	13 mg
Candy (per oz.)	
Ghirardelli Dark Chocolate	24 mg
Hershey's Milk Chocolate	4 mg

Dairy Products

Women with PMS symptoms should avoid dairy products. This always surprises women, because dairy products have traditionally been touted as one of the four basic food groups; many women count them as staples in their diet, eating large amounts of cheese, yogurt, milk, and cottage cheese.

Yet dairy products are extremely difficult for the body to digest; they can worsen the depression and fatigue that coexist in many women with PMS symptoms. This is because the body must use so much energy to break them down before they can be absorbed, assimilated, and finally utilized. All parts of dairy products are difficult to digest—the fat, the protein, and the milk sugar. Digesting dairy products demands hydrochloric acids, enzymes, and fat emulsifiers, which a stressed and tired woman may not produce in sufficient quantities.

Many women are specifically allergic to dairy products, and dairy products intensify allergy symptoms in general. Besides physical symptoms, food allergies can trigger PMS-related anxiety, mood swings, and even fatigue in susceptible women. I see this often in my patients who have emotionally-based anxiety symptoms or PMS-related anxiety coexisting with food allergies.

Users of dairy products often complain of allergy-based nasal congestion, sinus swelling, and postnasal drip. They can also suffer from digestive problems such as bloating, gas, and bowel changes, which intensify with menstruation. Intolerance to dairy products can hamper the absorption and assimilation of calcium, an important anxiety-relieving mineral.

Dairy products have many other unhealthy effects on a woman's body. The saturated fats in dairy products put women at higher risk of heart disease and cancer of the breast, uterus, and ovaries. Women on a high-fat diet also tend to accumulate excess weight more easily. Many dairy products, such as cheese, are high in salt as well as fat. Excessive use of these foods can increase the risk of high blood pressure and of bloating and fluid retention. Bloating can cause uncomfortable breast tenderness and abdominal swelling, particularly in the premenstrual period.

Women who have depended on dairy products for their calcium intake naturally wonder what alternative sources they should use. Women concerned about calcium intake can turn to many other good dietary sources of this essential nutrient, including beans, peas, soybeans, sesame seeds, soup stock made from chicken or fish bones, and green leafy vegetables.

For food preparation, rice, almond, flaxseed, sunflower seed, hemp and soy milk are excellent substitutes. These nondairy milks are readily available at health food stores. You can also use a supplement containing calcium, magnesium, and vitamin D to make sure your intake is sufficient.

Wheat and Other Gluten-Containing Grains

Women who have food allergies or PMS related mood problems may have difficulty digesting wheat. The protein in wheat, called gluten, is highly allergenic and difficult for the body to break down, absorb, and assimilate. Women with wheat intolerance are also prone to fatigue, depression, bloating, intestinal gas, and bowel changes, sinusitis and nasal congestion.

In my clinical experience, wheat consumption by women who tend towards anxiety and depression and are nutritionally sensitive can worsen emotional symptoms and fatigue. I have seen this happen with patients during the week or two before the onset of menses. Many menopausal women tolerate wheat poorly because their digestive tracts are beginning to show the wear and tear of aging and don't produce enough enzymes to handle wheat easily.

Women with allergies often find that wheat intensifies nasal and sinus congestion as well as fatigue. I also find that women with poor resistance and a tendency toward infections may need to eliminate wheat in order to boost their immune function. Because wheat is leavened with yeast, it should also be avoided by women with candida infections.

No matter what the cause of your PMS, if the symptoms are severe, you should probably eliminate wheat from your diet at least for one to three months during the early stages of recovery. Oats and rye, which also contain gluten, should be eliminated along with wheat. Good grain options for women with PMS include brown rice, millet, quinoa, buckwheat and amaranth.

Buckwheat is one of the least stressful grains for women with PMS and other hormone related health issues, probably because it is not commonly eaten in our society. Also, it is actually a grass, thus is not in the same plant family as wheat and other grains.

Many of these gluten-free grains are also used in breads, pastas and cereals and are available in many health food stores and some supermarkets. Women with PMS may find that they feel their best by eliminating gluten-containing grains like wheat and rye on an ongoing basis. If you want to include oatmeal in your diet, you can purchase gluten-free oatmeal that is available in health food stores and some supermarkets.

Alcohol

Women with moderate to severe PMS should avoid alcohol entirely or limit its use to occasional small amounts. Alcohol is a simple sugar, rapidly absorbed by the body. Like other sugars, alcohol increases hypoglycemia symptoms; excessive use can increase PMS related anxiety and mood swings. (See the preceding section on sugar for a thorough discussion of this process.) This can be particularly pronounced in women with PMS-related hypoglycemia.

Once alcohol has been absorbed and assimilated, it is primarily metabolized by the liver. This is a complex process requiring much work on the part of the body. Excessive intake of alcohol can overwhelm the liver's ability to process it, leading to toxic by-products that can themselves affect mood. Too much alcohol can also impede the body's ability to detoxify other chemicals—including drugs, hormones such as estrogen, and pesticides—that we take into our bodies by choice or through environmental contact.

As a result, toxic levels of these chemicals can build up in the body, worsening PMS. Excessive levels of estrogen seen in women with PMS, young women on birth control pills, and menopausal women on estrogen replacement therapy, have been linked to altered mood states and anxiety.

This can occur when the therapeutic estrogen dose prescribed by the physician is in excess of the body's needs.

Alcohol, an irritant to the liver as well as to other parts of the digestive tract, may be used by the body for immediate energy or stored in the liver or in the rest of the body as fat. Unfortunately, the liver cannot convert alcohol to a storage form of glucose.

As a result, the amount of fat stored in the liver increases with excessive alcohol use. Alcohol raises the liver enzyme level, leading to liver inflammation (or hepatitis). Eventually the chemical by-products of alcohol and the fat derived from alcohol can cause scarring and shrinkage of the liver, leading to functional impairment of the liver and cirrhosis.

In addition, alcohol irritates the lining of the upper digestive tract, including the esophagus, stomach, and upper part of the small intestine. It also causes irritation and inflammation of the pancreas. Over time, this can result in worsening of hypoglycemia and diabetes as well as impaired absorption and assimilation of essential nutrients from the small intestine. Certain of these nutrients, such as the B vitamins, are necessary to stabilize these conditions.

The nervous system is particularly susceptible to the deleterious effects of alcohol, which readily crosses the blood-brain barrier and actually destroys brain cells. Alcohol can cause psychological changes and profound behavioral in women who use it excessively. Symptoms include emotional upset, irrational anger, emotional outbursts, poor judgment, loss of memory, mental impairment, dizziness, poor coordination, and difficulty in walking.

Symptoms of emotional upset triggered by alcohol can also be caused by candida overgrowth, since candida thrives on the sugar in alcohol. Alcohol can thus promote a tendency toward chronic candida infections. Women with candida-related mood upset and fatigue need to avoid alcohol entirely. Furthermore, many women with allergies are sensitive to the yeast in alcohol, which worsens their allergic symptoms.

Given the preceding information on alcohol's adverse effects, I recommend that women with PMS symptoms use alcohol only very rarely. When used carefully—not exceeding 4 ounces of wine per day, 12 ounces of beer, or 1 ounce of hard liquor—alcohol can have a delightfully relaxing effect in women who have normal energy levels. It can make us more sociable and enhance the taste of food.

However, women who are particularly susceptible to the negative effects of alcohol shouldn't drink at all. If you entertain a great deal and enjoy social drinking, try non-alcoholic beverages. A nonalcoholic cocktail, such as mineral water with a twist of lime or lemon or a dash of bitters, is a good substitute. Some people enjoy and find that nonalcoholic beer tastes quite good. Light wine and beer also have a lower alcohol content than hard liquor, liqueurs, and regular wine.

Salt

Although salt does not specifically increase PMS, women should watch their salt intake carefully and avoid excessive intake for optimal health and well-being. Too much salt in the diet can cause many physical problems. It can worsen bloating and fluid retention, as well as increase high blood pressure, and is a risk factor in the development of osteoporosis in menopausal women. In addition, salt can deplete the body of potassium, a mineral necessary for healthy nervous system function.

Unfortunately, most processed foods contain large amounts of salt. Frozen and canned foods are often loaded with salt. In fact, one frozen-food entree can contribute as much as one-half tea-spoon of salt to your daily intake. Large amounts of salt are also commonly found in the American diet as table salt (sodium chloride), MSG (monosodium glutamate), and a variety of food additives.

Fast foods such as hamburgers, hot dogs, French fries, pizza, and tacos are loaded with salt and saturated fats. Common processed foods such as soups, potato chips, cheese, olives, salad dressings, and ketchup (to name only a few) are also very high in salt. To make matters worse, many people use too much salt while cooking and seasoning their meals.

For women of all ages, I recommend eliminating added salt in your meals. For flavor, use seasonings such as garlic, herbs, spices, and lemon juice. Avoid processed foods that are high in salt, including canned foods, olives, pickles, potato chips, tortilla chips, ketchup, and salad dressings. Learn to read labels and look for the word sodium (salt). If it appears high on the list of ingredients, don't buy the product. Many items in health food stores are labeled "no salt added." Some supermarkets offer "no added salt" foods in their diet or health food sections.

Summary Chart: Foods to Avoid or Minimize

Coffee
Tea (containing caffeine)
Chocolate
Soft drinks containing caffeine
Sugar
Alcohol
Dairy products
Wheat and gluten-containing grains
Salt

How to Cut Sugar Craving

Breaking the cycle of addiction to sugar is not easy. It is a particularly acute problem for women who have intellectually demanding jobs or hobbies (for example, reading or writing). The brain is a major user of the available sugar in the blood: after intense mental activity, the blood sugar level drops and the brain signals for more glucose. During the premenstrual period, the demand for sugar becomes even stronger.

Most women respond to the demand for sugar by going for quick energy sources such as fruit juice, chocolate, candy, cake, or cookies—anything sweet that's around the house. This works for the short term, but in the long run it causes an erratic, roller-coaster pattern in which the pancreas, liver and adrenals are throwing the blood sugar level back and forth from high to low.

It is far preferable to eat the more slowly metabolizing complex carbohydrates such as grains, legumes, and vegetables. All of these foods have a complex structure that is more slowly broken down in the digestive process. These causes the blood sugar level to rise slowly, peak slowly and fall slowly, stabilizing the woman's moods and cravings as well as her energy.

For many women it is enough to eat these complex carbohydrates during meals, but some women may need to eat them as between-meal snacks with additional protein or essential oils as well in order to keep their blood sugar levels stable. Gluten-free bread or crackers spread with sesame butter or tuna fish is a particularly good snack for this problem.

How to Beat Caffeine Addiction

If you drink three or four or more cups of coffee a day, you probably will not be able to quit abruptly because of the withdrawal headache caffeine causes. It's best to cut down by a half-cup or so a day. You can replace the coffee or tea with another warm drink, either herb tea or a roasted-grain beverage that tastes like coffee. If you drink herb teas, remember to drink a variety, because many herbs are strong substances, with untoward effects of their own if taken in excess.

Caffeine, like nicotine, is a work-drug for many people. If you have been depending on caffeine to help you work better, try meditation, repeating affirmations or exercise instead. See the chapters on stress and exercise.

If you depend on coffee to wake you up and help you stay alert, substitute ginger tea: Add two tablespoons of grated ginger root to 4 cups of water. Boil for five minutes and steep for fifteen minutes. This tea can be stored in the refrigerator and reheated.

How to Fight Chocolate Addiction

Chocolate addiction is basically sugar addiction, complicated by the fact that chocolate is a complex food, containing—in addition to sugar—fat, caffeine, mood elevators called theobromines and the mood-stabilizing mineral magnesium. To fight a severe chocolate addiction, replace the chocolate with carob which is in the legume family, high in calcium, and does not contain the addictive chemicals of chocolate. Or enjoy other healthy types of desserts and baked goods like oatmeal cookies, rice flour based shortbread, date and nut cookies, and desserts without added sugar. All of these products are available in health food stores.

In addition, use a multi-vitamin, multi-mineral complex that contains at least 400 to 500 mg magnesium, 50 mg B-complex, and 200 mcg chromium per day to reduce the chocolate cravings.

How to Get Eating Binges Under Control

The tendency towards binging and snacking, often on unhealthy sugary and fatty foods, is a real problem for many women with PMS. In my own medical practice, women have literally used my office as a confessional booth, telling me about the ice cream bars, chocolate cake, French fries, and potato chips that they find themselves unable to resist when PMS cravings are at their most intense.

There are several things you can do to reduce the tendency to binge. First of all, increase intake of fiber and fiber-rich foods, such as whole grain cereals, breads, crackers, and other baked goods. It is often helpful to combine them with a healthy omega-3 or omega-6 rich nut or seed butter like almond butter or sesame butter, or spread a little bit of water-packed tuna on a rice cracker with a small amount of low fat mayonnaise.

This combination of complex carbohydrates with essential oils and protein will help you blunt your appetite by stabilizing your blood sugar level and also because these foods digest more slowly.

In addition, salads with mixed greens, beans, hard-boiled eggs or tuna, soups, and cut up fresh raw vegetables like peppers, carrots, and celery are also bulky and filling. They help to reduce cravings as well as the desire to snack and binge. It is imperative that such snacks be available at work to avoid eating the pastries that are often set out with the coffee or from running to the candy machine in midafternoon.

Chew your food slowly and thoroughly. Women who binge tend to bolt down their food without chewing well. This places additional stress on the digestive tract, for it has to work hard to break down and assimilate food. Do not eat your big meal at night, for your body processes food inefficiently while you are sleeping, and you will tend to gain weight. Eat your main meal at noon and dine lightly in the evening. Keep a calendar in the kitchen and mark a star or an X for cheating to remind you each day of your goals. Make a tape of your own voice with your affirmations such as "I want to eat only at mealtimes. I do not feel a need to binge. I enjoy the beauty of my lovely figure." All of these methods will help program your mind and body chemistry for success.

How to Lessen Fatigue and Improve Stamina

Many women with PMS complain of feeling spaced-out, tired, and lethargic. Standard pick-me-ups like coffee, tea, or sweets only worsen the problem, but there are some herbs that help build stamina and energy in the long run. I have found the following to be helpful for women with PMS-related fatigue.

Tyrosine. This amino acid combines with iodine within the thyroid gland to form the thyroid hormone thyroxine. Thyroxine controls metabolic rate, and regulates carbohydrate and fat metabolism. Women whose protein intake is low or who can't absorb and assimilate protein due to digestive problems, may lack sufficient tyrosine in their diets. These women may have borderline low thyroid levels which can be remedied by increasing their protein intake.

Tyrosine may also be taken as a dietary supplement. Generally, 500 to 1500 milligrams of tyrosine per day may be used. It is best to take tyrosine with a meal high in carbohydrates. Women using monamine oxidase (MAO) inhibitor drugs for the treatment of depression should avoid taking tyrosine as should those diagnosed with melanoma.

Phenylalanine. Within body tissues, tyrosine is manufactured using another amino acid, phenylalanine. This essential amino acid must be acquired through the diet. Good food sources include fish, poultry, red meat, soybeans, almonds, lentils, lima beans, chickpeas, and sesame seeds. It may also be taken as a supplement, with 500 to 2,000 milligrams as the usual therapeutic dosage. Be sure to start at the lower end of this range, increasing gradually. Phenylalanine is a natural antidepressant and pain killer, but can also cause jitteriness and nervousness when used in too high a dose. It should be avoided by women using monoamine oxidase inhibitor drugs for depression.

Vitamin B-complex. This complex consists of eleven vitamin B factors which work together to perform such metabolic functions as glucose metabolism, stabilization of brain chemistry, and inactivation of estrogen. Heavy menstrual bleeding can result in anemia due to low levels of iron in the blood, deficiency of three B-complex vitamins: folic acid, pyridoxine (vitamin B6), and vitamin B12. Vitamin B6 helps reduce PMS-related mood swings, fatigue, food cravings, and fluid retention. The B-complex vitamins are usually found together in beans and whole grains. I recommend 25-100 mg of B vitamins per day taken as a supplement.

Magnesium. Magnesium deficiency is seen in women suffering from PMS. Medical studies have shown low red blood cell magnesium during the second half of the menstrual cycle in affected women. Magnesium supplements can benefit women with emotional stress, anxiety, and insomnia. Good food sources include dark leafy vegetables, beans and peas, raw nuts and seeds, tofu, avocado, raisins, dried figs, millet, and other grains. I recommend 400-500 mg of magnesium as a supplement per day.

Potassium. Potassium helps maintain the body's fluid balance and helps prevent PMS bloating symptoms. Abundant food sources include fruits, vegetables, beans and peas, seeds and nuts, starches, and whole grains.

How to Combat Periodic Weight Gain

If your weight gain is due to fluid retention (the most common reason in women with PMS) several solutions may be helpful. Use a mildly diuretic tea like uva ursi and parsley. Eat foods that are high in potassium and have a diuretic effect such as cucumbers, melons and bananas. Be sure to eliminate added salt from your diet as salt worsens fluid retention and bloating considerably. Throw away your salt shaker, and eat as many fresh fruits and vegetables as possible.

Avoid processed foods such as ketchup, mustard, and salad dressings which are high in salt. Be sure to read labels of all processed foods to make sure they have no or very low levels of added salt (less than 150 mg per serving). Also avoid fried and fatty foods. I have found that these foods worsen bloating. Women with an allergic tendency should take special care to avoid wheat and dairy products, which can worsen bloating and weight gain. The addition of digestive enzymes like bromelian 500-1000mg two to three times a day or pancreatin 300-600 mg two to three times a day can help to relieve bloating due to allergic inflammation.

Also, make sure that your bowels are working properly, so that you don't reabsorb fluids and waste products that should be eliminated from the body. This can cause excess weight gain. Women who have problems with constipation should be sure to include bran in their diets. One to eight tablespoons per day should suffice. Bran can be mixed with soup or water or baked into muffins.

8

Planning and Preparing Meals

Healthy and delicious meals can provide you with many essential nutrients to support your health and wellness during your active reproductive years. This is particularly important if your goal is to use a healthy diet and good nutrition to relieve and prevent PMS symptoms. A successful PMS relief diet will provide important hormonal support and along with many additional health benefits.

Happily, just by making some simple dietary modifications, you can make a major difference in your health. In this chapter I have included many beneficial and delicious PMS relieving menus that you can add to your roster. Over the years, these meal planning guidelines have helped many of my patients implement their own self-help programs, and their feedback has been very positive.

Many patients have noted an immediate improvement in their health and well-being and found the new foods delicious and satisfying. I hope these dietary suggestions will be helpful to you, too. This healthful diet can also benefit and be enjoyed by your entire family.

However, no one diet fits the needs of all different body types. Because of this I have included menus and delicious recipes for women who prefer a vegetarian emphasis, high complex carbohydrate diet as well as dishes and entrees for women who feel their best on a high protein, meat-based diet. All of these meal plans and the recipes in the next chapter contain ingredients that are very beneficial for women who are dealing with issues related to PMS as well as other health issues. In addition, the high stress ingredients that can worsen your symptoms have been eliminated. Let's now look at PMS relief meal plans for breakfast, lunch and dinner.

Morning seems to be the hardest part of the day for most of us. There always seems to be too much to do and not enough time. As a result on weekdays many women skip breakfast entirely. Others eat foods like doughnuts and coffee in hopes of getting quick energy. On weekends, when most of us take time off, we eat more traditional breakfasts consisting of - coffee, milk, white toast, cheese, butter, sweet rolls, sugar laden cereals, white flour pancakes and waffles. Any one of these scenarios can wreak havoc for the PMS sufferer.

Breakfast is the most important meal of the day. Eating a nourishing breakfast can provide the energy and sense of well-being that is so important to getting your tasks for the day done. Surprisingly enough, I've found that for most of my patients, even though breakfast is often the worst-planned meal of the day, it is also the easiest meal to restructure, because it's the meal that is most under their control. They do not have to contend with the limited choices available in a restaurant or cafeteria or the social pressure of eating with friends. Your goal should be a breakfast that is quick and easy to prepare, delicious, and useful in minimizing PMS symptoms.

Breakfast Menus

These breakfast menus have been developed to help reduce and prevent symptoms of PMS. All the dishes contain high levels of the essential nutrients that women with these problems need; the recipes call for no high-stress ingredients. You can use these as idea generators for your own meal planning.

Breakfast has been one of the easiest meals for my patients to restructure along healthier lines. It tends to be a smaller and simpler meal. You may want to make healthful dietary changes in your breakfast first and then move on to lunch and dinner.

Flax shake with protein powder
and fresh fruit
~~~~~~~~~~~~~~

Blueberry and spirulina smoothie
~~~~~~~~~~~~~~

Millet cereal with raisins and
cinnamon
Nondairy yogurt
Chamomile tea
~~~~~~~~~~~~~~

Rice and flaxseed pancakes
Banana
Vanilla nondairy milk
~~~~~~~~~~~~~~

Oatmeal with raspberries
Chamomile tea
~~~~~~~~~~~~~~

Nondairy yogurt with granola
and ground flaxseed
Peppermint tea
~~~~~~~~~~~~~~

Scarmbled eggs with turkey
bacon
Lemon ginger tea
Orange slices
~~~~~~~~~~~~~~

Omelette with chicken sausage
Roasted grain beverage (coffee
substitute)
Apple slices
~~~~~~~~~~~~~~

Lunch and Dinner Menus

Here is a variety of menus you can choose from when planning your meals. You can use these menu plans or as idea generators to fit your own taste and needs. These dishes contain many nutritious and healthful ingredients for PMS relief. Use these menus as helpful guidelines throughout the entire month. Your nutritional status on a day-by-day basis determines in part how likely you are to have PMS symptoms. These dishes should help to diminish the severity of your symptoms because they eliminate high-stress foods.

Soup Meals
Split pea soup
Corn muffins
Fresh applesauce
~~~~~~~~~~~~~

Chicken and wild rice soup
Cole slaw
Millet bread with flax oil
~~~~~~~~~~~~~

Vegetable soup with brown rice
Steamed kale
Baked potato with flax oil
Apple slices
~~~~~~~~~~~~~

Lentil soup
Herbed brown rice
Broccoli with lemon
~~~~~~~~~~~~~

Tomato soup
Potato salad with low-fat mayonnaise
Celery and carrot sticks
~~~~~~~~~~~~~

Salad Meals
Spinach salad with turkey bacon or tofu
Corn muffins with flax oil
Orange slices
~~~~~~~~~~~~~

Beet salad with goat cheese
Rice crackers with fresh fruit preserves
~~~~~~~~~~~~~

Romaine salad with grilled salmon
Gluten-free bread and olive oil dip
~~~~~~~~~~~~~

Low-fat potato salad
Cole slaw
Hard boiled eggs
Melon slices
~~~~~~~~~~~~~

Mixed Vegetable Salad with Kidney Beans
Baked yam

Meat Meals

Poached salmon with lemon
Herbed brown rice
Steamed carrots with honey

~~~~~~~~~~~~~~

Roasted chicken with herbs
Baked potato with flax oil
Broccoli with lemon

~~~~~~~~~~~~~~

Broiled trout with dill
Mixed green salad with vinaigrette
Green peas and onions
Apple slices

~~~~~~~~~~~~~~

Grilled shrimp with olive oil and
lemon
Wild rice
Steamed kale

~~~~~~~~~~~~~~

One-Dish Vegetable Meals

Vegetarian tacos with black beans,
brown rice, avocados, tomatoes,
lettuce and low-salt salsa

~~~~~~~~~~~~~~

Stir-fry with mixed vegetables,
brown rice and tofu
Orange slices

~~~~~~~~~~~~~~

Pasta with tomato sauce, broccoli,
carrots, olive oil and garlic
Green salad with vinaigrette

~~~~~~~~~~~~~~

Hummus dip
Eggplant dip (babaganoush)
Mixed raw vegetable slices
including carrots, red bell peppers,
and radishes

~~~~~~~~~~~~~~

Brown rice and almond tabouli
Mixed olives
Melon slices

~~~~~~~~~~~~~~

9

The Women's Diet Cookbook

During my college and medical school years, I entertained often. My friends and I all enjoyed cooking and sharing meals together. I suffered from very bad PMS symptoms and menstrual cramps during this time and didn't realize that all of the rich dishes I prepared with lots of cheese, butter, cream, sherry and Madeira and tons of rich sugary desserts were greatly contributing to my symptoms.

During my postgraduate medical training, I finally began to piece together the nutritional basis for many of my PMS symptoms. When I finally realized how badly I had been sabotaging myself, I was shocked: the wonderful lingering rich meals were directly connected to my pain, bloating, and bad moods.

I was determined to improve my dietary habits and eliminate my PMS symptoms. All of the fat-and sugar-based cooking went out the window and I started over with learning to prepare a more whole food dietary approach, eating foods that were close to the earth such as more fresh vegetables, whole grains, legumes and free range meats.

I began to explore Asian cooking and tomato-based Indian curries and dal made from lentils, all of which eliminated the need to cook with a lot of milk products, sugar, salt and other high stress ingredients. As I learned the basics of a more fresh and whole food cuisine, I began adapting my individual recipes by adding ingredients that corrected PMS and eliminating any that worsened it. Then I began substituting low-stress ingredients for high-stress ingredients in other recipes, especially recipes for desserts, which for me were among the hardest things to give up.

Eventually, without my really planning it, a cuisine evolved that used only foods that were good for women. I began sharing my recipes with my patients, and their enthusiastic responses (and requests for a cookbook) got me started on this book.

When it was time to test the recipes for the book, I did all the cooking myself and enjoyed it very much. Having a house full of happy tasters reminded me of my school days—except that this time the food was good for us and easy to prepare. It was very gratifying to see everyone, including men and even young children, enjoying the food created initially for women with PMS. So I don't think you have to worry about sharing your diet with your family and friends

Since no one diet approach works for all women, I have included in this chapter both whole grain, complex carbohydrate-based entrees as well as meat-based, protein rich dishes, depending on the type of diet that makes you feel your best. Both types of entrees, however, will benefit PMS symptoms by eliminating wheat, dairy products, sugar and other high stress ingredients. Best of all, they are all made with delicious, nutrient-rich healthy ingredients!

Adapting the Women's Diet for Pregnancy or Menopause

The Women's Diet is excellent for pregnancy and menopause if it is adapted slightly to take into account the special dietary needs of those periods in our lives. Calcium is especially important for pregnant women and nursing mothers because the developing baby puts additional demands on the mother's own supply; and for women in menopause because the decrease in hormone levels tends to cause demineralization of the bones. The pregnant woman also needs large amounts of iron in her diet because her blood volume is expanding tremendously, creating a tendency toward anemia.

For both pregnant women and women in menopause, sea vegetables such as dulse and kelp are important because their rich supply of iodine and trace minerals provides nutrients essential for normal endocrine function (especially of the thyroid). For more specific information, consult books on these topics.

Breakfast Recipes

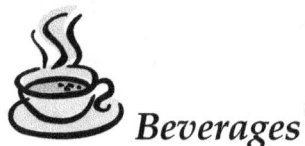 *Beverages*

These drinks are made with therapeutic herbal teas, power smoothies that are rich in fruits, raw seeds, nuts, protein powder, green foods and non dairy milk that are recommended for preventing and treating your symptoms. The ingredients contain high levels of essential nutrients that help regulate your hormonal balance and eliminate your symptoms of PMS. You can enjoy these beverages throughout the month, and not just during your symptom time, as their high mineral and other nutrient content is beneficial for the entire body.

Relaxant Herb Tea   **Serves 2**

2 cups water
1 teaspoon chamomile leaves
1 teaspoon peppermint leaves
1 teaspoon honey (if desired)

Bring the water to a boil. Place herbs in water and stir. Turn heat to low and simmer for 15 minutes.

Peppermint and chamomile are both muscle relaxants and antispasmodic herbs, so they can provide relief of pain and cramping caused by PMS and menstrual cramps. They also help calm the mood.

Ginger Tea   **Serves 4**

Ginger makes a warming, delicious tea and is beneficial to your circulation. It is also a powerful anti-inflammatory herb. If the tea is too strong add more water.

5 cups water
3 tablespoons ginger coarsely chopped
½ lemon (optional)
Honey (or other sweetener, to taste)

Add ginger to the water in a cooking pot. Bring to a boil and then turn heat to low. Steep for 15 or 20 minutes. Squeeze lemon into tea and serve with honey or your favorite sweetener.

Blueberry Pomegranate Smoothie   **Serves 2**

¼ cup nondairy yogurt, unsweetened
¾ cup pomegranate juice
1 cup blueberries, fresh or frozen
1 tablespoon ground flaxseed
1 banana

Combine all ingredients in a blender. Puree until smooth and serve.

Raspberry Flax Smoothie   **Serves 2**

This creamy smoothie makes a great breakfast. Flaxseed oil one is my favorite foods. It is both delicious and rich in healthy omega-3 fatty acids. It also adds extra creaminess to the smoothie.

1 cup rice milk
⅔ cup raspberries – fresh or frozen
1 heaping tablespoon rice protein powder
1 tablespoon flaxseed oil
2 bananas, sliced

Combine all ingredients in a blender. Puree until smooth and serve.

Delicious Green Drink   **Serves 1**

½ cup Concord grape juice
¼ cup water
1 tablespoon ground flaxseed
½ teaspoon chlorella powder
½ teaspoon spirulina powder

Mix all ingredients together in a glass or puree in a blender.

Heavenly Strawberry Coconut Smoothie   **Serves 2**

This drink fits its name! It is absolutely scrumptious as well as good for you. If you don't have a high-speed blender and you are using whole raw cashews I recommend that you chop them up beforehand. Otherwise, raw cashew butter is a good substitute.

1 cup coconut drink (Coconut Dream brand preferred)
1 cup strawberries – fresh or frozen
1 tablespoon raw coconut flour
1 tablespoon raw cashews (about cashews 10-15)
1 banana, sliced

Combine all ingredients in a blender. Puree until smooth and serve.

Simple Flax Smoothie   **Serves 2**

Flaxseed is not only a tasty addition to smoothies but it is also very nutritious. Flaxseed is high in essential fatty acids, calcium, magnesium, and potassium.

1 cup vanilla nondairy milk
2 tablespoons ground flaxseed
1 banana

Combine all ingredients in a blender. Blend until smooth and serve.

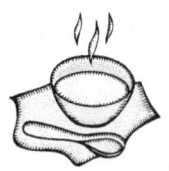 *Healthy, Quick Breakfasts*

Most American breakfasts include wheat and dairy products, such as milk, butter, wheat toast, wheat and sugar based cereals with milk, sweet rolls, and other wheat-based pastries. Sugar is also another common ingredient found in many prepackaged breakfast foods. Dairy products, wheat and sugar can worsen the symptoms of PMS.

I have included in this section both whole grain, complex carbohydrate based entrees as well as protein-rich dishes, depending on the type of diet that makes you feel your best. Both types of entrees, however, will benefit PMS symptoms by eliminating wheat, dairy products and sugar at breakfast.

The vegetarian dishes are based on ground flaxseed, soy, and gluten-free grains, all of which can be useful in reducing your symptoms. Gluten is the protein found in wheat that can trigger symptoms of bloating, digestive disturbances, and fatigue. Gluten-free oats are now available in health food stores, some supermarkets and on the Internet. The protein-rich entrees have been created using eggs and healthy breakfast meats.

Quinoa Cereal with Blueberries   **Serves 2**

1 ½ cups cooked quinoa
1 cup nondairy milk
½ cup blueberries
2 teaspoons honey or other sweetener

Combine quinoa and nondairy milk in a saucepan. Simmer for 5 minutes. Stir in honey and garnish with raspberries.

Quinoa with Prunes

Serves 2

This is one of my all-time favorite hot cereals. The plums are delicious and add a nice texture. Quinoa is a small, protein rich grain. When cooked the grains are small and fluffy. I recommend making a pot of quinoa the night before.

1 ½ cups cooked quinoa
1 cup nondairy milk
4-6 dried prunes, chopped
2 tablespoons flaxseed oil
2 teaspoons xylitol, honey, or maple syrup (if using unsweetened milk)
Pinch of salt (optional)

In a saucepan combine quinoa, nondairy milk, salt, and dried plums. Heat thoroughly and simmer on low heat for 5-10 minutes until plums have softened. Serve with flaxseed oil and sweetener.

Maple Cinnamon Oatmeal

Serves 2

1 cup gluten-free quick oats
1 ¾ cups water
1-2 tablespoons flaxseed oil
2 teaspoons maple syrup
Pinch of cinnamon (to taste)
Pinch of salt

Boil water in a saucepan. Add gluten-free oats and reduce to medium heat. Cook for one minute and stir. Cover, and remove oatmeal from heat. Serve in 2-3 minutes.

Stir in maple syrup, flaxseed oil, cinnamon and salt.

Strawberries and Cream Oatmeal   **Serves 2**

1 cup gluten-free quick oats
½ cup strawberries, chopped
½ nondairy milk
1 ¼ cups water
1-2 tablespoons flaxseed oil
2 teaspoons honey or stevia
Pinch of salt (optional)

Bring water and nondairy milk to a boil in a saucepan. Add gluten-free oats and reduce to medium heat. Cook for one minute and stir. Cover, and remove oatmeal from heat. Serve in 2-3 minutes. Stir in sweetener, flaxseed oil, salt and top with strawberries.

Flaxseed Pancakes   **Makes 8 pancakes (serves 2-4)**

Xylitol is an excellent sugar substitute for cooking and baking that can be found at most health food stores. Xylitol is easy to use because it has a 1:1 ratio with sugar. Yet, this product has 40% fewer calories than sugar and is beneficial for your teeth and gums.

1 cup gluten-free flour
1 cup unsweetened rice milk
1 egg
2 tablespoons xylitol
1 tablespoon ground flaxseed
1 teaspoon baking powder
½ teaspoon baking soda
¼ teaspoon salt
3 tablespoons almond oil, set aside 1 tbsp. for cooking
Maple syrup (optional)
Fruit jam (optional)

Mix the dry and wet ingredients in separate bowls. Combine all the ingredients and mix thoroughly. Cook on medium heat and use a small amount of oil to grease the pan if needed. When pancakes bubble in the center flip and cook for 1-2 minutes until cooked thoroughly. Serve with maple syrup or all-fruit jam. Delicious!

Apple Almond Muffins

The cinnamon and apples in these muffins makes the kitchen smell delicious and welcoming. If you are eating a nut-free diet simply omit the nuts.

2 cups rice flour
1 apple, diced (Granny Smith apple preferred)
½ cup applesauce
6 packets of Truvia (equal to ¼ cup sugar)
1 tablespoon honey
½ cup water
1 egg
3 tablespoons safflower oil
⅓ cup chopped almonds
1 teaspoon cinnamon
¼ teaspoon nutmeg
1 teaspoon baking powder
½ teaspoon baking soda
Pinch of salt

Preheat oven to 400 degrees. Mix all dry ingredients and wet ingredients separately. Combine and pour a large spoonful (approximately a heaping tablespoon) into each muffin cup. I recommend using baking cups for this recipe.

Bake for 20 minutes until cooked through.

Pumpkin Muffins

Makes 14-18 muffins

1 ½ cups rice flour
½ teaspoon baking powder
½ teaspoon baking soda
1 cup pumpkin
1 teaspoon cinnamon
¼ teaspoon nutmeg
¼ cup chopped almonds (optional)
3 tablespoons molasses
3 tablespoons safflower oil
½ cup raisins
2 eggs
½ cup nondairy milk
1 teaspoon vanilla extract
Pinch of salt

Preheat oven to 400 degrees. Line a muffin tin with paper muffin cups.

Combine all dry ingredients and mix thoroughly. In a separate bowl beat the two eggs and then combine the remainder of the wet ingredients. Add the wet ingredients to the dry and mix thoroughly.

Fill muffin cups ⅔ with the batter. Cook for 18-20 minutes or until thoroughly cooked.

Egg and Sausage Scramble   **Serves 2**

4 eggs
4 turkey breakfast sausages
2 slices of gluten-free toast
Salt and pepper (optional)
2 teaspoons olive oil
Serve with ½ cup applesauce

Warm a frying pan on medium heat and add olive oil. Beat egg gently in a small bowl and set aside. Chop the sausages into small pieces - this will help them to cook faster. Add sausages to the pan and cook for several minutes until sausages are brown. Turn heat to low and add eggs to the pan and scramble with the sausage. Add a pinch of salt and pepper. Serve with toast and applesauce.

Bake for 20-25 minutes until cooked through.

Red Pepper and Sausage Wrap   **Serves 2**

2 brown rice tortillas
½ cup red pepper, diced
⅓ cup onion, diced
3 eggs, beaten
2 turkey breakfast sausages, cut into small pieces
1 tablespoon olive oil
Salt and pepper – generous pinch

In a frying pan on medium heat the olive oil. Add the sausage and cook until lightly browned. Add the onions and red peppers and cook until onions begin to soften, about 2 minutes. Next, add eggs and salt and pepper. Let eggs sit until they begin to cook slightly and then scramble.

Lightly warm the tortillas and put the egg scramble into the tortillas. Top the eggs with one tablespoon of salsa.

Spinach and Tomato Scramble   **Serves 2**

The Parmesan cheese added as a garnish provides a delightful saltiness and tang to this dish.

4 eggs, beaten
1 tablespoon water
2 tablespoons diced onion
¼ tomato, chopped
12 spinach leaves, chopped
1 tablespoon olive oil
Salt and pepper (optional)
Parmesan cheese - or soy Parmesan (optional)

Beat the 4 eggs together with 1 tablespoon water. Preheat the frying pan on medium heat and add 1 tablespoon olive oil. Add onion and cook for about 3 minutes until onions are translucent. Next add eggs, spinach and tomato. Let sit for about 15 seconds and then start to scramble with your spatula. Sprinkle on a small amount of Parmesan cheese, add a pinch of salt and pepper and serve

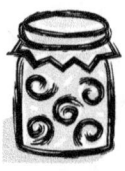 *Spreads and Sauces*

These spreads and sauces contain highly concentrated levels of ingredients that help to reduce PMS related symptoms and even help to relieve congestion. Serve with rice cakes, crackers, corn bread, or even spread on a banana for a delicious treat.

Fresh Applesauce   Serves 2

2 ½ apples
½ cup fresh apple juice
½ teaspoon cinnamon
½ teaspoon ginger

Peel apples and cut into quarters; remove cores. Combine all ingredients in a food processor. Blend until smooth.

Sesame-Tofu Spread   Serves 4

¼ cup soft tofu
¼ cup raw sesame butter
¼ cup honey

Combine all ingredients in a blender. Serve with rice cakes or crackers.

Lunch and Dinner Recipes

These high-nutrient, healthful lunch and dinner dishes are designed to help prevent and relieve your symptoms. The ingredients do not include red meat, dairy products, or wheat, all of which can worsen your symptoms. Mix and match these dishes as you please. You might combine soups and salads or whole grains, legumes and vegetables for a complete vegetarian emphasis or meat-based meal, depending on your needs for carbohydrates and protein.

The main course dishes are all extremely healthful for women with PMS. You can enjoy these dishes particularly during the second half of your menstrual cycle when your symptoms are worse, but for optimal health and well-being, I recommend their use all month long.

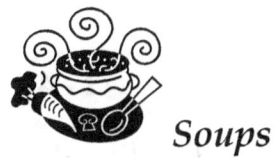 *Soups*

Split Pea Soup   **Serves 4**

¾ cup split peas
5 cups low-sodium chicken broth
⅔ cup carrot, chopped
¾ cup onion, diced
Tamari soy sauce – to taste (optional)

Bring the water to a boil and add the split peas, onion, carrots, and chicken broth. Reduce heat to low and simmer for 50-60 minutes, stirring occasionally. If water begins to cook off add up to an extra cup of water. Add a dash of tamari soy sauce for a saltier flavor.

Black Bean Soup

Serves 4

This recipe is easy and makes a delicious, filling soup.

1 can black beans (14 ounce), rinsed
5 cups low-sodium vegetable broth
1 cup onion, diced
⅔ cup carrot, chopped
⅔ cup red pepper, chopped
¼ teaspoon cumin
Tamari soy sauce – to taste (optional)

Bring the water to a boil and add all ingredients. Reduce heat to low and simmer for 30 minutes, stirring occasionally. If water begins to cook off add up to an extra cup of water. Add a dash of tamari soy sauce for a saltier flavor.

Chicken Rice Soup

Serves 4-6

Few things make me feel better than a bowl of homemade chicken rice soup. I have an easy tip to add extra flavor to your soup: If you used the meat from a roasted, skin-on chicken you can add some of the skin to the soup while it is cooking. This will add depth and richness to your soup. Remove the skin when the soup has finished cooking.

6 cups low-sodium chicken broth
⅔ cup carrot
1 cup celery, diced
1 cup cooked chicken, diced
⅔ cup onion, diced
⅔ cup brown rice, cooked
Tamari soy sauce – to taste (optional)

Bring water to a boil and add all ingredients. Reduce heat to low and simmer for 30 minutes, stirring occasionally. If water begins to cook off add up to an extra cup of water. Add a dash of tamari soy sauce for a saltier flavor.

Butternut Squash Soup **Serves 4**

This soup has been a long-time favorite of mine. I adore the light, creamy texture. Adding maple syrup enhances the natural sweetness of the squash.

½ onion, diced
1 cup low-sodium chicken broth
2 cups pureed butternut squash - fresh or frozen (fresh is preferred)
½ teaspoon cinnamon
1½ cups nondairy milk
2 teaspoons maple syrup
1 tablespoon safflower oil
½-¾ teaspoon salt

In a large saucepan heat the oil on medium heat. Add the onion and cook until translucent. Add the butternut squash, chicken broth, cinnamon and salt. Mix well and simmer for 5 minutes. Add nondairy milk and maple syrup. Simmer on low heat for ten minutes. Stir frequently while cooking the soup.

Optional: To make extra creamy, blend the soup when it has finished cooking. Wait for the soup to cool before blending.

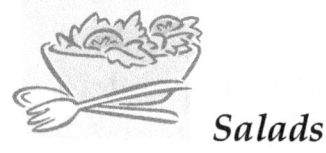

Salads

Zingy Watercress Salad   Serves 4

I enjoy the refreshing bitterness of watercress. This salad pairs well with green apple. Watercress has a strong flavor and a little goes a long way.

1 cup watercress, coarsely chopped
4 cups butter lettuce (or other soft lettuce), coarsely chopped
2 teaspoons scallions, finely chopped
½ green apple, chopped
1 ounce goat cheese, crumbled
Vinaigrette dressing

In a large bowl toss the watercress, butter lettuce, green onion, and apple together with the vinaigrette dressing (to taste). On top of the salad crumble the goat cheese.

.

Caesar Salad   Serves 2-4

I love Caesar salads. They have been my favorite salad for years! The crispy romaine lettuce and creamy dressing is a perfect match. I like to use anchovies because they are delicious in this salad and also full of healthy anti-inflammatory oils. I prefer the filets packed in olive oil.

1 head of romaine lettuce, chopped – about 6 cups
4 tablespoons light Caesar dressing
4 anchovy filets, chopped
⅔ cup gluten-free croutons
1 ½ teaspoons grated Parmesan cheese
1 cup roast chicken, cubed (optional)

In a large mixing bowl pour Caesar's dressing over lettuce. Mix well so that leaves are evenly coated with dressing. Add croutons, Parmesan cheese, anchovies, and toss well. Top with roasted chicken and serve.

Classic Spinach Salad   **Serves 4**

My tip for cooking great turkey bacon is to cook it on medium-low heat. It takes a few extra minutes but is definitely worth it!

1 bunch of spinach, approximately 6 cups
4 slices of turkey bacon, cooked crisp and crumbled
2 eggs, sliced or chopped
½ cup red pepper, chopped
¼ red onion, sliced very thin
¾ cup mushrooms, sliced thin
Balsamic vinaigrette dressing

In a large bowl place the bacon, egg, red pepper, onion, and mushrooms on top of the spinach. Mix in the dressing and toss before serving.

Scrumptious Veggie Salad   **Serves 4-6**

This is one of my favorite salads! It pairs wonderfully with soups and sandwiches.

1 head red lettuce, chopped into bite size pieces
1 large tomato, chopped
2 green onions, sliced
6 mushrooms, sliced
¾ cup kidney beans
1 avocado, sliced
¼ cup sunflower seeds
Vinaigrette dressing (to taste)

Combine all ingredients except for avocado in a large salad bowl. Mix in vinaigrette dressing and top with avocado slices before serving.

Radicchio and Orange Salad   **Serves 4-6**

This is a sophisticated and delicious salad. I love salads with "extras" such as fruit or a little bit of goat cheese.

6 cups salad greens
½ radicchio, sliced thin
⅓ red onion, sliced very thin
3 ounces goat cheese
1 medium sized orange, peeled and cut into bite size segments
Orange vinaigrette

In a large bowl combine salad greens, radicchio, onion, and oranges. Pour vinaigrette dressing (to taste) over salad and toss. Add goat cheese before serving.

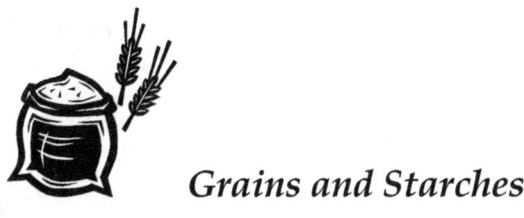 *Grains and Starches*

Wild Rice   Serves 2

⅔ cup wild rice
2 ½ cups water
½ teaspoon salt

Wash rice with cold water. Combine all ingredients in a cooking pot and bring to a rapid boil. Turn flame to low, cover, and cook without stirring (about 45 minutes) until rice is tender but not mushy. Uncover and fluff with a fork. Cook an additional 5 minutes, and then serve.

Kasha   Serves 4

1 cup kasha (buckwheat groats)
3 ¼ cups water
Pinch of salt

Bring ingredients to a boil, lower heat, and simmer for 25 minutes or until soft. The grains should be fluffy, like rice.

For breakfast, blend in blender with water until creamy. Add almond milk, sesame milk, or sunflower milk, and cinnamon, apple butter, raisins, or berries.

Delicious Baked Sweet Potato   Serves 4

4 sweet potatoes
1 teaspoon olive oil
1 tablespoon flax oil for each potato

Preheat oven to 400° F. Wash the potatoes, then rub with olive oil. Bake for 45 to 60 minutes, or until soft when pierced with a fork. Garnish with flax oil. Honey, maple syrup, or chopped raw pecans may also be used.

Baked Potato **Serves 4**

4 russet or Idaho potatoes
2 teaspoons olive oil
1 tablespoon flax oil for each potato

Preheat oven to 400° F. Wash the potatoes, rub them with olive oil, and bake for 45 to 60 minutes, or until soft when pierced with a fork. Garnish with flax oil. Other garnishes can include chopped green onions, soy cheese, and salsa.

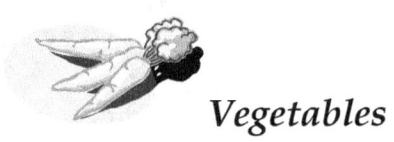

Vegetables

Kale with Lemon   Serves 4

Kale is one of my favorite vegetables and it also has terrific health benefits for women since it is a good source of calcium and other essential nutrients like lutein that supports the health of your eyes.

1 bunch of kale
1 lemon, cut into quarters
Soy sauce

Rinse kale well and remove stems. Steam for 5-6 minutes or until leaves wilt and are tender. Dress lightly with soy sauce and lemon juice.

Simple Steamed Cabbage   Serves 4

1 small head cabbage, quartered
1 teaspoon chopped parsley
1 teaspoon olive oil
Pinch of salt (optional)

Steam cabbage until tender. Sprinkle with olive oil and parsley.

Jessica's Favorite Broccoli   Serves 4

1 pound broccoli
1 tablespoons flax oil
Pinch of salt (optional)
Squeeze of lemon

Cut the broccoli into small florets; steam until tender. Squeeze lemon juice over broccoli and add the flax oil. Mix and serve.

Cauliflower with Flax Oil

Serves 4

1 medium head cauliflower
2 tablespoons flax oil
Pinch of salt (optional)

Break the cauliflower into small florets. Steam until tender. Toss with flax oil and salt.

Roasted Rosemary Potatoes

Serves 4-6

I love roasted potatoes! This is a wonderful potato recipe that I like to make when I serve roasted chicken.

4 cups red potatoes – about 4 or 5 large red potatoes
1 tablespoon dried rosemary, crushed
3 tablespoons of olive oil
2 garlic cloves, minced
¼ teaspoon pepper (optional)
Pinch of salt

Preheat oven to 400 degrees. Cut potatoes into bite size pieces and put into plastic bag. Add olive oil, rosemary, garlic, and pepper to bag. Close bag and shake to coat all of the potato pieces.

Line a baking tray with foil and put potatoes on to tray. Arrange evenly in one layer. Sprinkle salt onto potatoes and bake for 30-35 minutes until brown and cooked through. During cooking stir the potatoes once if desired.

Honey Carrots Serves 4

This is one of my favorite side dishes. The warm honey brings out the natural sweetness of the carrots.

3 cups carrots, sliced thin
1 teaspoon honey
1 teaspoon almond oil
Pinch of salt (optional)

Cut carrots into thin slices and steam for 6-8 minutes, or until tender. Using the same saucepan pour out the cooking water and on low heat add the honey and oil and mix well. Add carrots and mix all ingredients together. Add a pinch of salt before serving.

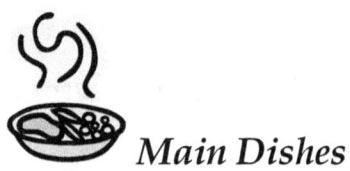 *Main Dishes*

Mega Greens Rice Bowl   **Serves 4**

This dish is a satisfying way to get a large serving of healthy greens. A delicious sauce is Organicville's Island Teriyaki (organicvillefoods.com). Their sauce is made with agave nectar instead of cane sugar.

4 cups kale, cut into bite size pieces (about ½ bunch)
3 cups baby bok choy, chopped
1 cup of white mushrooms, sliced
1 carrot, finely chopped
8 ounces of tofu, cubed
3 cups cooked brown rice - ¾ cup rice per person
Teriyaki sauce – soy sauce - gomasio

Steam the carrots for 4 minutes and then add the kale, bok choy, mushrooms, and tofu. Steam for 5 minutes. Serve in a deep bowl over rice with your choice of sauce.

Good sauces for this dish include teriyaki sauce and soy sauce. A little bit of lemon juice and gomasio also works well.

Teriyaki Tofu Wrap   **Serves 2**

The tofu and teriyaki flavors blend delightfully with the vegetables. This is a light and delicious wrap.

2 brown rice tortillas
6 ounces of baked tofu, cubed or sliced
¼ red pepper, sliced thinly
2 radishes, sliced thinly
1 cup salad greens
½ cup sprouts
2 tablespoons teriyaki sauce

Lightly heat up the tortilla until soft. Layer the vegetables inside and top with the tofu. Lightly pour the sauce on top. Wrap and serve.

Summertime Veggie Pasta   **Serves 4**

This light pasta is one of my favorite dishes to eat during the summer. The pasta and sauce are light but filling. It's a dish that I love to share to share with friends.

1 box quinoa elbow pasta (8 ounce box)
½ onion, diced
2 cans Italian seasoned diced tomatoes
1 can garbanzo beans
1 carrot, shredded
1½ cups cooked Brussels sprouts or broccoli
½ teaspoon dried basil
2 teaspoons olive oil
Pinch of pepper
Pinch of salt (optional)

Cook pasta according to package directions. In a saucepan on medium heat add olive oil and onions. Sautee until onions are translucent. Add remainder of ingredients and bring to a simmer. Cook on low heat for 10 minutes. Combine the cooked noodles with the sauce.

Eggplant Parmesan   **Serves 4-6**

I love eggplant Parmesan. It is a rich and extremely delicious entree. This version, while wonderful, takes a little more time and has a few more steps than most of my entrees. Even though I use substitutions for the cheese, the dish is still very rich and I recommend saving it for a special occasion or party. You will wow your guests with how tasty it is! My favorite cheese alternative is by Follow Your Heart. Their products can be found in health food stores or at followyourheart.com

1 eggplant, cut into ⅓ - ½ inch slices (peeling is optional)
2 eggs, beaten
1 ¼ cups gluten-free breadcrumbs
3 cups of pasta sauce, tomato and basil flavor
8 ounces of mozzarella cheese, shredded
⅓ cup Parmesan or soy Parmesan cheese, grated
¼ cup olive oil - divided

Arrange the eggplant slices in a colander or on a rack placed over the sink. Sprinkle all of the slices generously with salt and let stand 30 minutes; the eggplant slices will release water. Rinse and pat dry. Next, dip each slice in the beaten egg and coat with breadcrumbs.

Heat a portion of the olive oil in a skillet over medium heat. Cook the eggplant until golden on each side, about 2-3 minutes. If necessary, reduce the heat to medium-low. Repeat until all of the eggplant is cooked.

Preheat the oven 350°. Arrange half the eggplant slices on the bottom of a lightly oiled baking dish (a 9x9 or 9x12 pan works well). Spread half of the pasta sauce on top. Sprinkle with half of the mozzarella and half of the Parmesan cheese. Repeat with the next layer.

Bake 25-30 minutes or until mixture is bubbly.

Parmesan Chicken Pasta **Serves 4**

This dish is a crowd pleaser that I often serve when I have friends over. The garnish of Parmesan cheese adds a delightful tanginess that rounds out the dish perfectly.

6 cups gluten-free pasta, cooked
1 ½ cups roasted chicken, cubed
⅔ cup diced carrots
⅔ cup diced red onion
½ onion, diced
1 small tomato, finely chopped
3 cups broccoli, chopped into bite size pieces
⅔ cup chicken broth (recommended) or water
1 teaspoon dried basil
1 tablespoon olive oil
Soy Parmesan cheese or regular, grated (to taste)
Generous pinch of pepper
Pinch of salt (optional)

In a frying pan on medium heat add the olive oil. Add the onion and sauté until onion begin to turn translucent. Add all vegetables except tomatoes and cook for 1-2 minutes. Add chicken broth, chicken, tomatoes, basil, and pepper. Turn heat to low, cover and simmer for 5-7 minutes or until broth has cooked down. Add more broth if needed.

Add the sauce to the pasta. Serve with Parmesan cheese.

The PMS Cure   105

Turkey Bolognese

Serves 2-4

This dish cooks up quickly and is very satisfying. This is a versatile recipe. You can add all kinds of vegetables and it will taste great.

½ lb. ground turkey
2 cans of diced tomatoes
1 can tomato paste
½ onion, diced
1 carrot, diced
1 zucchini, diced
1 teaspoon basil
1 teaspoon oregano
1 tablespoon olive oil
¼ teaspoon salt (optional)
½ teaspoon pepper (optional)
Water (optional)

Heat pan on medium and add olive oil. Add onion and sauté until translucent. Add turkey and all herbs and spices. Cook until turkey has browned and cooked thoroughly. Add tomatoes, tomato paste, carrots, and zucchini. Cook on low heat for 12-15 minutes. If sauce is too thick add a small amount of water until desired consistency is reached. Serve over brown rice spaghetti.

Simple Broiled Tuna

Serves 4

4 fillets of tuna, 4 ounces each
2 teaspoons olive oil
Squeeze of lemon juice
Pinch of salt

Baste the tuna fillets with oil; then sprinkle with lemon juice. Place tuna in a broiler pan and broil until the level of doneness that you prefer (rare or well-done).

Simple Steamed Salmon   **Serves 4**

4 fillets of salmon, 4 ounces each
1 cup water
Squeeze of lemon

Combine water and lemon juice in a steamer. Place salmon fillets in streamer basket. Cook to the level of doneness that you prefer.

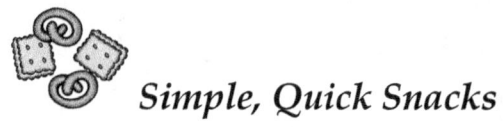 *Simple, Quick Snacks*

Trail Mix   Makes ¾ cup

¼ cup raw unsalted pumpkin seeds
¼ cup raw unsalted sunflower seeds
¼ cup raisins

Combine and store in a container in the refrigerator. This trail mix is very high in essential fatty acids, calcium, magnesium, and iron. I use it for a snack food to replace stressful and unhealthy sugar-based sweets and chocolate. It is a great mix to take on trips, and I eat it often for breakfast.

Rice Cakes with Nut Butter and Jam   Serves 2

4 unsalted rice cakes
2 tablespoons raw almond butter
2 tablespoons fruit preserves (no sugar added)

Spread rice cakes with almond butter and fruit preserves for a quick snack.

Herbal tea makes a good accompaniment.

Rice Cakes with Tuna Fish   Serves 2

4 unsalted rice cakes
4 ounces tuna fish
1 teaspoon low-calorie mayonnaise

Spread rice cakes with tuna fish and mayonnaise.

This is an excellent high-protein, high-carbohydrate snack.

Apple with Almond Butter   **Serves 2**

1 apple, sliced
1 tablespoon raw almond butter

Spread almond butter on thin apple slices.

Banana with Sesame Butter   **Serves 2**

1 banana, halved
1 tablespoon raw sesame butter

Spread sesame butter on each half of a ripe banana.

10

Vitamins and Minerals for PMS

There are a number of vitamins, minerals, herbs and other nutrient that are important in overcoming PMS. If you shop from the PMS shopping list and eat a wide variety of foods, you will get many beneficial nutrients. But if you have moderate to severe PMS symptoms, the use of a therapeutic nutritional supplement program is also very important.

It is very helpful to use the nutritional supplements that I discuss in this chapter and also emphasize the foods that are high in these beneficial substances. For example, a woman with acne might want to eat more carrots; a woman with cramps more leafy green vegetables; a woman with heavy bleeding more buckwheat and citrus fruits, in addition to their nutritional supplement program.

Let's now look at the vitamins, minerals, herbs and other nutrients that are beneficial for relieving the symptoms of PMS.

Vitamins and Minerals and What They Do

Vitamin A. Vitamin A helps to improve the health of your skin. It is useful in suppressing premenstrual acne and oily skin. There are two types of vitamin A. Vitamin A from animal sources such as fish oil is stored in the liver and can be toxic if taken in too large a dose (greater than 25,000 international units [I.U.] a day for several months).

Beta-carotene, a precursor of vitamin A found in plant sources, is more easily absorbed upon ingestion. It is not toxin in large amounts. A single carrot can have as much as 10,000 I.U. Some other good food sources of vitamin A are listed in the food charts.

Some Food Sources for Vitamin A

Adult recommended daily allowance: 5,000 I.U.
Therapeutic requirements for PMS: 13,000 - 40,000 I.U.

Carrots	Beet greens
Butternut squash	Bok choy
Salmon	Broccoli
Dandelion greens	Sweet red peppers
Hubbard squash	Apricots
Sweet potatoes	Romaine lettuce
Turnip greens	Peaches
Kale	Asparagus
Mustard greens	Butter lettuce

Pycnogenol and Isoflavones have significant effects on the physiology of premenstrual women. Studies show that pycnogenol, which is derived from pine bark or grape seeds, reduces bloating, fluid retention, and breast tenderness at 50 mg once or twice daily.

Isoflavones such as genistein and daidzein are natural sources of plant estrogen found in soybeans and other soy products. These weak, estrogen-like chemicals help to modulate the effects of the more powerful estrogens made by the body. They help to reduce mood swings, fluid retention, and headaches in dosages from 50 to 100 mg per day.

Vitamin B-Complex. The vitamin B-complex consists of eleven factors that work together to perform important metabolic functions, including glucose metabolism, inactivation of estrogen by the liver, and stabilization of brain chemistry. The B-complex vitamins are usually found together in foods such as whole grains, brewer's yeast, liver, and legumes, but the relative amounts of the individual factors vary considerably from food to food.

Emotional stress causes loss of the water-soluble B vitamins from the body. Fatigue and irritability can be the result.

My recommended therapeutic dosages for PMS for some of the important B vitamins are:

Thiamine (vitamin B1)	25-50 mg
Riboflavin (vitamin B2)	25-50 mg
Niacin (vitamin B3)	50 mg
Biotin	500 mcg
Pantothenic acid (vitamin B5)	50 mg
Pyridoxine (vitamin B6)	50 mg
Para-aminobenzoic acid	50 mg
Choline	50 mg
Inositol	50 mg
Cyanocobalamin (vitamin B12)	100-750 mcg
Folic acid	400-800 mcg

Choline and Inositol. Among the B vitamins, choline, inositol and B6 are known to be of particular importance in preventing PMS. Choline and inositol enhance the liver's ability to break down fatty foods and fat-soluble hormones such as estrogen. Inositol is also a central nervous system tranquilizer and may help to calm premenstrual anxiety and irritability. Inositol and choline are found in high amounts in soybean, wheat germ, bran, and corn.

Vitamin B6. Daily doses of between 50 - 100 mg can help to regulate many premenstrual symptoms including mood swings, breast tenderness fluid retention, irritability, bloating, sugar craving, and fatigue. However, doses above this level can be toxic and should be avoided. (Research done at UCLA and other institutions noted this.) Vitamin B6 levels may decrease in women using birth control pills.

If you take individual B vitamins, it's important to take the rest of the complex, too.

Some Food Sources of Vitamin B6

Adult recommended daily allowance: 2 milligrams
Therapeutic requirements for PMS: 50 - 100 milligrams

Salmon	Rye flour
Chicken	Brown rice
Tuna	Broccoli
Soybeans	Asparagus
Rice Bran	Wheat germ
Kale	Brussels sprouts
Buckwheat flour	Beet greens
Navy beans	Green peas
Lentils	Sunflower seeds
Lima beans	Sweet potatoes
Pinto beans	Cauliflower
Black-eyed peas	Brewer's yeast
Shrimp	Leeks
Whole wheat flour	

Vitamin C. Vitamin C is an important antioxidant and ant-stress vitamin. It is necessary for adrenal cortical hormone synthesis and for immune function. It also has an antihistamine effect, which can help women whose allergies worsen before their periods. Vitamin C also helps to reduce symptoms of emotional stress and fatigue by supporting adrenal functions. I prefer mineral buffered vitamin C for best results.

Some Food Sources of Vitamin C

Adult recommended daily allowance: 45 milligrams
Therapeutic requirements for PMS: 500 milligrams - 3 grams

Sweet red peppers	Lemons
Brussels sprouts	Turnips
Collard greens	Peas
Sorrel	Red raspberries
Kale	Blackberries
Green peppers	Lima beans
Strawberries	Chard leaves
Lamb's-quarters	Tomatoes
Kohlrabi	Spinach
Cauliflower	Pineapples
Mustard greens	Sweet potatoes
Oranges	Potatoes
Grapefruit	Blueberries
Cabbage	Mung bean sprouts
Rutabagas	Bananas
Salmon	Chicken

Vitamin E. Early research linked adequate levels of vitamin E with fertility in rats. This suggested that vitamin E has a powerful effect on the hormonal system. This has been corroborated in the last fifteen years by clinical testing.

In a Johns Hopkins University Medical School study, vitamin E was found to be quite effective in reducing PMS symptoms including the anxiety, irritability, depression, and food cravings, were decreased by as much as twenty-five to thirty percent in women using 400 I.U. of vitamin E daily. Vitamin E was also found to reduce PMS-related breast tenderness or mastalgia in 600 I.U. dosage studies done at several institutions including Johns Hopkins University Medical School.

Some Food Sources of Vitamin E

Adult recommended daily allowance: 12 - 15 I.U.
Therapeutic requirements for PMS: 400 - 1600 I.U.

Wheat germ oil	Peanut oil
Walnut oil	Broccoli
Sunflower oil	Brussels sprouts
Sweet potato	Apples
Safflower oil	Rye
Turnip greens	Peas
Beet greens	Corn
Leeks	Parsnips
Wheat germ	Blackberries
Asparagus	Cornmeal
Corn oil	Wheat
Sesame oil	

Calcium. Adequate calcium intake helps to reduce menstrual pain, as well as PMS related moodiness and fluid retention. The beneficial effect of calcium on PMS symptoms was reported in a study in the *American Journal of Obstetrics and Gynecology.* Calcium helps maintain normal muscle tone and helps prevent cramps and pain. It is present in the foods listed below.

Some Food Sources of Calcium

Adult recommended daily allowance: 800 – 1000 milligrams
Therapeutic requirements for PMS: 800 - 1000 milligrams

Collard leaves	Broccoli
Salmon	Tofu
Shrimp	Okra
Blackstrap molasses	Dandelion greens
Sesame seeds	Masa harina
Bok choy	Soybeans
Kale	Carob flour
Mustard greens	Rutabagas

Magnesium. Research done at UCLA Medical School, found that women with PMS have decreased magnesium levels. Magnesium helps to relieve menstrual cramps and control premenstrual sugar craving. It also helps to normalize glucose metabolism and stabilize moods by effecting brain chemistry. Magnesium actually optimizes the amount of usable calcium in your system by increasing calcium absorption. Conversely, calcium can interfere with magnesium absorption. The usual recommendation of calcium is twice as much as magnesium, but for the PMS patient, the ratio can be reversed for the first six to twelve months of treatment. A specific form of magnesium, magnesium aspartate, has also been found to decrease fatigue, a real problem for some women with PMS.

Some Food Sources of Magnesium

Adult recommended daily allowance: 400 - 500 milligrams
Therapeutic requirements for PMS: 500 milligrams (in supplement)

Soybeans	Wheat berries	Pecans
Black-eyed peas	Sesame seeds	Beet greens
White beans	Lentils	Oatmeal
Peanut butter	Chicken	Shrimp
Dandelion greens	Parsnips	Peas
Cauliflower	Lima beans	Cashews
Red beans	Rye flour	Beets
Buckwheat	Turnips	Tofu
Salmon	Brown rice	Corn
Turnip greens	Sweet potatoes	Pistachios
Cornmeal	Kale	Barley
Whole wheat flour	Almonds	Asparagus
Millet snap beans	Mushrooms	Cabbage
Brussels sprouts	Green peppers	Collards
Sunflower seeds	Celery	Broccoli
Summer squash	Onions	Peanuts
Filberts (Hazelnuts)	Carrots	Lettuce
Mustard greens	Tomatoes	Walnuts

Zinc and Manganese. Zinc is important in conjunction with vitamins A and C for the control of acne. It competes with copper for binding sites and displaces copper in the body. An adequate dietary supply of zinc is important because an overabundance of copper can increase moodiness and increase levels of estrogen. Much of the world's soil is zinc-depleted making it more difficult to obtain zinc in the diet.

The previously cited study in the *American Journal of Obstetrics and Gynecology* also examined the role of manganese in relieving PMS symptoms. The study found that decreased manganese intake worsened the tendency toward PMS mood and pain symptoms. I recommend 2 – 5 mg of manganese per day.

Some Food Sources of Zinc

Adult recommended daily allowance: 15 milligrams
Therapeutic requirements for PMS: 15 to 25 milligrams

Soy meal	Buckwheat
Wheat bran	Oatmeal
Wheat germ	Brown rice
Chicken	Millet
Rice bran	Soy protein
Black-eyed peas	Apples
Whole wheat flour	Corn
Wheat berries	Cabbage
Green peas	Onions
Cornmeal	Whole wheat bread
Garbanzos	Peanut butter
Lentils	Carrots
Lima beans	Rye bread
Soy flour	

Herbs That Help PMS

Herbs, the traditional treatment for illness for thousands of years, were originally tested not by modern methods but empirically, as people tried them and noted their effects. The body of knowledge thus acquired is still available to us today, and many of my patients prefer plant-based remedies to drugs.

Herbs can be looked upon as a form of extended nutrition. Since they are plants, they can make up part of your regular diet when used in small amounts. They help to balance the body chemistry and correct disease symptoms due to nutritional factors. For example, cold symptoms can occur when people eat an abundance of high-stress foods. Medicinal herbs such as burdock and kudzu plus a light diet of vegetables and whole grains can help to correct the imbalance and relieve the cold symptoms.

If you are under stress and feel anxious, herbs such as valerian and chamomile can help to stabilize your mood because they calm and tranquilize the central nervous system. They can also help relieve PMS-related insomnia. Herbs that have been used traditionally to relieve hormonal problems in women include black cohosh, licorice, blessed thistle, sarsaparilla, red raspberry leaf, wild yam, and gotu kola. For decades, herbalists have observed that these herbs to be beneficial for PMS.

I use herbs in my medical practice as a means of balancing the diet and optimizing the nutritional intake. For example, in Traditional Chinese Medicine, acne is thought to be due to a predominantly yin or expansive diet that is high in sugar and fat. This can be corrected by balancing the diet with herbs such as dandelion root or burdock root, which are bitter and highly concentrated in their mineral content.

In contrast, menstrual cramps are thought to be due to an excess of yang foods such as meat and salt. These are foods that have a contracting effect on the body. For some women, this can be countered by chewing a yin root like ginger, which causes dilation of the blood vessels and relaxation.

Some herbs contain high concentrations of nutrients such as calcium, magnesium, and potassium, which Western medical research has found to be important in controlling a variety of PMS symptoms. Good sources of these minerals include dandelion, raspberry leaf, parsley, kelp, and alfalfa.

Herbs should be used in small amounts and taken with your meals either in capsule form or in a tea. If you prefer to make a tea, simply empty the capsule into a cup of boiling water and let it seep for a few minutes. Do not drink more than one or two cups of the tea per day. There are some contraindications to the use of herbs. Herbs should not be used if you are currently on a hormone prescribed for you by your doctor.

All foods have the potential for causing distress in some people. Herbs are no exception. They should be discontinued immediately if you notice nausea, vomiting, or diarrhea upon using. These are the most common symptoms of intolerance. The herbs in my formula are all recommended as being safe for human consumption, but some women seem to have a specific intolerance for various foods, including herbs. If you notice any symptoms that make you uncomfortable after using the herbs, discontinue them immediately.

Essential Fatty Acids for PMS

Essential fatty acids are important nutrients for women with PMS. They consist of two types of special fats, called linoleic acid (omega-6 family) and alpha-linolenic acid (omega-3 family). These fats must be supplied in your diet daily, either from foods or nutritional supplements.

Essential fatty acids are found in the membrane structure of all cells. They are required for normal development and function of the brain, eyes, inner ear, adrenal glands, and reproductive tract. The essential oils are needed to synthesize prostaglandins I and III. These hormone-like chemicals help decrease the risk of heart disease, boost immune function, decrease menstrual cramps, and reduce PMS symptoms.

An important essential oil for PMS treatment is evening primrose oil (omega-6 family). Clinical studies have shown as much as a 65 percent reduction in PMS symptoms, particularly fluid retention, breast tenderness, and mood swings. Evening primrose oil contains gamma-linolenic acid (GLA), and essential fatty acid, which is a precursor to prostaglandin type 1. Other good (and less expensive) sources of GLA include borage oil and black currant oil. Flaxseeds and chia seeds contain omega-3 fatty acids, which are precursors to the synthesis of series-3 prostaglandin. It is important to include these oils in your diet, also. Vitamin B6 and magnesium, as well as several other nutrients, are needed to convert linoleic acid to GLA resulting in producing the beneficial prostaglandins. Thus, these nutrients should be included in your PMS program also.

Evening primrose oil, borage oil, and black currant oil are taken by capsule, while flaxseed oil is also delicious for food preparation. Both the seeds and their pressed oil become rancid when exposed to light and air. They must be packed in opaque containers and kept in the refrigerator. Good quality flaxseed oil is available in health food stores.

An additional benefit is that both flax and chia seeds are the best sources of both essential fatty acids (linoleic acid and alpha-linolenic acid). Essential fatty acids are extremely beneficial for women, but they must be derived from dietary sources because they cannot be produced by the body.

Flaxseed oil is golden, rich, delicious, and extremely high in linoleic and alpha-linolenic acid (which comprise about 80 percent of its total content). Flaxseed oil has a wonderful flavor and can be used as a butter replacement. Flaxseed oil (and all other essential oils) should never be heated or used in cooking as it affects their chemical properties. Add these oils to cooked foods as flavoring. I recommend using one to two tablespoons of flaxseed oil each day. Another great option is ground flaxseeds which can also be purchased in health food stores or online.

A research study done at the University of Michigan Medical School found that women who used ground flaxseeds had more frequent and regular ovulations and menstrual periods since the lignans found in the flaxseeds helped to trigger progesterone production. I recommend using two to four tablespoons stirred into hot cereal, smoothies or shakes.

Omega-3 fatty acids are also found in abundance in fish, which are rich sources of eicospentaenoic acid (EPA) and docosahexaenoic acid (DHA). The best source is cold water, high-fat fish such as salmon, tuna, rainbow trout, mackerel, and eel. Because of the high levels of mercury found in many fish, however, it is best to limit fish intake to no more than once or twice a week and use fish oil capsules instead. Omega-3 fatty acid intake of 1500 to 3000 mg. total per day is a good therapeutic dosage for PMS and menstrual cramps, too. Vegetarians can use algae (seaweed) sources of EPA and DHA.

Linoleic àcid (omega-6 family) is found in many seeds and seed oils. Good sources include safflower, sunflower, corn, sesame seed, and wheat germ oil. Many women prefer to use raw sesame seeds, sunflower seeds, and wheat germ to obtain the oils. The average healthy adult requires four teaspoons of essential oils in their diet per day. For optimal results, use these oils along with vitamin E, which also helps prevent rancidity of the oils in the body.

An excellent combination of essential fatty acids for women with PMS would include a combination of flaxseed oil, borage oil, and vitamin E (to prevent rancidity). This can be put together easily by buying the essential oils in your local health food store.

Amino Acids for PMS

Several amino can be very useful in the treatment of PMS related emotional symptoms and sleep disturbances. .

5-hydroxytryptophan. This amino acid derivative can be converted within the body to serotonin, the neurotransmitter that regulates mood swings, sleep disturbances, and food cravings, all commonly seed with PMS. By normalizing brain chemistry, 5-hydroxytryptophan (also called 5-http) is an effective PMS treatment. Take 50 to 100 mg once a day and, before bedtime, if desired.

Tyrosine. This amino acid is a natural mood elevator and antidepressant. It supports healthy thyroid function and helps to promote mental and emotional energy, optimism and zest for living in women who tend towards PMS depression by its beneficial effect on brain chemistry. Dosage is 1000 mg per day with a protein meal or snack.

Nutritional Supplements for Women with PMS

Good dietary habits are crucial for control of your PMS symptoms. But for many women, the use of nutritional supplements is important in order to achieve high levels of the essential nutrients needed to heal PMS. On the following pages is a sample of the vitamins and minerals as well as their dosages that can be used as a foundation for your program.

You can also add the other nutrients like flaxseed oil and fish oil that I have discussed in this chapter to fill out your program. You may find it easier to implement your program if you start with one of the better quality multi-nutrient products for women that are available in health food stores and through the internet and then add the remaining essential nutrients.

Remember that all women differ somewhat in their nutritional needs. If you do take the recommended vitamin or herbal supplements, I usually advise that you start with one-fourth to one-half the dose recommended in this book and work your way up slowly to the higher dosage, if needed. You may find that you do best with slightly more or less of certain ingredients.

I recommend that patients take their supplements with meals or at least a snack. Very rarely, a woman will have a digestive reaction to supplements, such as nausea or indigestion. If this happens, stop all supplements; then resume using them, adding one at a time, until you find the offending nutrient. Eliminate from your program any nutrient to which you have a reaction. If you have any specific questions, ask a health-care professional who is knowledgeable about nutrition.

Vitamins

Beta-carotene	5,000-50,000 I.U.
Vitamin A	3,500-10,000 I.U.
Vitamin B1 (thiamine)	25-100 mg
Vitamin B2	25-100 mg
Niacinamide	25-100 mg
Pantothenic acid	25-100 mg
Vitamin B6 (pyridoxine HC1)	50-100 mg
Folic acid	400-800 mcg
Biotin	200-500 mcg
Vitamin B12	100-750 mcg
Choline bitartrate	25-100 mg
Inositol	25-100 mg
PABA (para-aminobenzoic acid)	25-100 mg
Vitamin C (as mixed mineral ascorbates)	500-2000 mg
Vitamin D (cholecalciferol)	1000 I.U.
Vitamin E	400-1,000 I.U.

Minerals

Calcium (amino acid chelate)	400-1,000 mg
Magnesium	400-1,000 mg
Iodine	150 mcg
Iron (amino acid chelate)	18 mg
Copper	2.0 mg
Zinc	15-25 mg
Manganese	10 mg
Potassium	50-300 mg
Selenium	200 mcg
Chromium	100-200 mcg
Citrus bioflavonoids	800-1,500 mg
Borage oil	1,000-2,000 mg
Flaxseed oil	1-2 tbsp
Grape seed extract	50-100 mg

Summary Chart For Nutritional Supplements

I want to end this section by summarizing the nutritional supplements that you can take to help eliminate your PMS symptoms. These include:

1. **Vitamins and Minerals** - Vitamin A, Pycnogenol or Grape seed extract, Isoflavones, Vitamin B-Complex, Choline, Inositol, Vitamin B6, Vitamin C, Vitamin E, Calcium, Magnesium, Manganese and Zinc

2. **Herbs** – Valerian, chamomile, black cohosh, licorice, blessed thistle, sarsaparilla, red raspberry leaf, wild yam, gotu kola, dandelion, burdock root, ginger, raspberry leaf, parsley, kelp, and alfalfa

3. **Essential Fatty Acids** - Linoleic acid (omega-6 family) and alpha-linolenic acid (omega-3 family). The best sources of omega-6 fatty acids are evening primrose oil, borage oil, and black currant oil. The best source of omega-3 fatty acids are flaxseed oil and fish oil (EPA and DHA) from cold water, high-fat fish such as salmon, tuna, rainbow trout, mackerel, and eel

4. **Amino Acids** - 5-hydroxytryptophan and tyrosine

11

How to Reduce the Stress in Your Life

Women with PMS seem to be especially susceptible to environmental stress during the premenstrual period. Little irritations that normally wouldn't both them assume monumental importance. They become anxious, irritable, or angry at the world around them. Unfortunately, this emotional sensitivity is very common, affecting 80 to 90 percent of women with PMS.

I remember as a teenager hearing for the first time negative and joking comments about PMS. These comments often meant that a woman with PMS was being irritable and difficult. They also reflected the underlying cultural belief that women are innately unstable and mercurial, victims of their fluctuating chemistry.

This was the attitude that many women have complained to me about when seeking help through their medical providers. Women with PMS have tended to be treated with mood altering drugs or birth control pills. There has been little awareness of the role that nutrition, stress and other environmental factors play in triggering PMS mood and other symptoms.

We know now that the emotional stress symptoms of PMS are the result of a combination of factors. They are a response to many physical, environmental, and mental stresses. We also see that the fact that they are common does not mean that they are normal. What it does mean is that a lot of women have poor living habits. As we have seen, the symptoms of PMS can be greatly corrected with proper nutrition. With a physician's help, they can also be corrected by medications such as progesterone and the anti-prostaglandin drugs. But it is also very important to learn to manage social stress.

If your metabolism is already burdened chemically and renders you hypersensitive to cyclical changes in your hormones, it is important not to add to the problem by setting up a stressful personal environment. The questions in the PMS Workbook are an indication of how much stress there is in your life. Most of the women I see in my medical practice feel that they could do better. They feel that they could find ways to improve the quality of their environment. Even women who are completely happy with their professional and personal lives feel that they could learn to manage stress better. They have become tired of feeling extremely angry, anxious, or irritable during their premenstrual period.

Many of my patients have asked me about techniques for coping better with stress. Over the last nine years, I have worked out a strategy that seems to work. I send some women for counseling or psychotherapy, but the majority are looking for practical ways to manage stress on their own. They want to take responsibility for learning to handle their own problem, looking at their methods of dealing with stress, learning techniques to improve their habits and then practicing these techniques to improve their habits and then practicing these techniques on a regular basis. I find this self-help way to be the most effective of all.

The Physiology of Stress

Your reaction to stress is partly determined by the sensitivity of your autonomic nervous system. The nervous system consists of the brain, the spinal cord, and the peripheral nerves. It is divided by function into two parts: the voluntary nervous system and the involuntary (or autonomic) nervous system.

The voluntary nervous system manages activity in the conscious domain. For example, if you place your hand on a hot stove, pain fibers will trigger a response that is sent to the brain. The brain sends back an immediate response telling you to move your hand away before you burn yourself. You then pull your hand away, fast.

The autonomic nervous system regulates functions that the average person is usually unaware of, such as the circulation of the blood, muscle tension, pulse rate, respiration, and glandular function. The autonomic nervous system is divided into two parts that oppose and complement each other.

They are called the sympathetic and parasympathetic nervous systems, and they control the upper and lower limits of your physiology. For example, if excitement speeds up the heart rate too much, it is the parasympathetic nervous system's job to act as a control circuit and slow it down. If the heart slows down too much, then it is the sympathetic nervous system's job to speed it up.

Many women with PMS have overactive sympathetic nervous systems that are much worse during the second half of their cycle. An easily triggered sympathetic nervous system is fine if you are driving your car on the expressway on Saturday night and need to be on the lookout for drunken drivers. Your muscles tense and your blood vessels constrict so you can react to an emergency.

The problem with many women who have PMS is that their sympathetic nervous systems are always in a state of readiness to react to a crisis. This puts them in a constant state of tension or "fight or flight." They tend to react to small stresses the same way they react to real emergencies. Their adrenal glands increase their output of adrenaline and cortisone, adjusting the body chemistry to meet the crisis. Their hearts speed up, their pulses race, and their neck and shoulder muscles tense. The energy that accumulates in the body to meet this "emergency" must then be discharged, and it is. They yell at the children or they kick the dog and their systems come into balance once again.

Macro-Stress. Two types of stress have a significant impact on people's health: major life changes and small everyday irritants. Major life changes include such important events as marriage, divorce, birth of a child, and loss of a job. Other events may be totally outside of your control but can affect you just as strongly. These include the death of a parent or an automobile accident for which you are not at fault.

Human beings can adapt to change only up to a certain point without it taking a toll on their health. Even happy situations like the birth of a child mean making accommodations in your life. They take energy and require a period of adjustment.

When more than one important stress occurs in a short period of time, the effects are cumulative. This idea was developed by Dr. Thomas Holmes and his co-workers at the University of Washington Medical School. Holmes developed the Life Change Index based on a system of points: the more serious the stress, the more points were assigned to it. Thus the death of a spouse was given 100 points and considered to be much more traumatic than a change in a person's work hours, which was given only 20 points. Major life changes during a two-year period were totaled.

A score of 300 points or more indicated a serious major life stress. A person with such a high score was shown to be at extremely high risk for major illness. A person with a score between 200 and 299 was thought to be at medium risk and a person scoring under 200 points at low risk.

Few of my patients date the onset of their PMS to major life changes, but all agree that major life changes, when they occurred, worsened their symptoms.

If you have not already answered the questions in the Major Stress Evaluation (based on the Holmes Life Change Index), it would be a good idea to do that now.

Micro-Stress. While the Life Change Index is very useful in evaluating the seriousness of major changes, it is unable to assess each person's individual reaction pattern. For example, the loss of a job can be a very serious handicap and is undoubtedly a stress for everyone. However, one person might respond to it with illness and depression, while another would take it as a challenge for personal growth. Perhaps more significant in determining your resiliency in dealing with stress is how you manage little everyday irritations or micro-stresses. These can include a flat tire, missing a bus, being late for an appointment, a child's crying, overcooking a casserole, and a multitude of other happenings.

We each have our own list of "hot spots" that seem to exasperate us out of proportion to the incident itself. The micro-stresses in themselves may be insignificant, but these small incidents add up. On a daily basis they can be responsible for more wear and tear than the large and dramatic life changes that Dr. Holmes describes.

It will help you to become aware of how you deal these irritations. Does tension build up in your body? Does your breath become shallow as you become more upset, or do you begin deep breathing and exercising at the first sign of stress? Do you meditate to calm your mind? Many of my patients do not recognize their own early signs of stress. They are not aware that they are upset until the feelings become very strong. Then they smoke, eat too much, take pills, or become cranky and irritable. For most of us, effective stress management is something that has to be learned.

It is important that you evaluate your own areas of micro-stress. If you have not already taken the test, turn back and do it now. If you have already taken it, it would be a good idea to go back over it for a moment.

What Stress Does to Your Body

Now that you have evaluated the areas in your life that produce stress, it is important to see how stress localizes in your body. In most people it causes tension in the muscles which is perceived as a tightness, soreness, or aching. The chronic tension obstructs the blood flow to that area of the body, cutting off the flow of oxygen to the tissues. The cells do not receive the nutrients that they need to function properly.

As a result, the muscles function at a low energy level. Toxic wastes can't be disposed of efficiently and lactic acid accumulates. This leads to fatigue. These aches and pains are your body's signal to you that you need to relax. The test that I have included will help you remember the places in your body where tension is most likely to accumulate.

Try to remember also whether there are particular tasks that seem to make your muscles ache. Do they occur at any particular time of day?

Managing Stress

Stress can be managed in three ways:

- going to a qualified professional for counseling

- restructuring your environment to make it less stressful

- learning relaxation techniques

Going to a Qualified Counselor

This can be a great help for those who feel they need it and have the resources. But since this is a self-help book, you will be functioning as your own counselor. You will need to look within and see what areas you would like to change in your life to make it more pleasant. Only a person who is stuck with the need to be a victim will say, "There's nothing I can do." Obviously that isn't you, or you wouldn't be using this book.

Restructuring Your Environment

We all tend to become oblivious to our surroundings at times. We see them, yet we don't see them. If you go through your day like a robot, simply doing your tasks and enduring discomfort, it's time now to stop and ask yourself what you can do to improve your life.

Physical Environment. Have you made your work and home attractive with pictures, plants, or personal accessories? Surrounding yourself with soothing colors and soft music helps you deal with stress.

Job. If you dislike your job, try to find another. You might want to take night courses or weekend seminars to prepare yourself for a different field or job level. Even if you can only do this slowly, it will give you something positive to focus on and you'll be learning something that you enjoy. Discuss problems on the job with your boss to see if you can make it a more enjoyable experience.

Work more slowly during the times of day when you begin to drag. Pace yourself, knowing when you tend to experience fatigue. Upgrade your energy during this time by closing your office door or going into your bedroom to listen to a relaxation tape, do deep breathing or meditate. (The specific techniques given in the next section take a few minutes and can increase your energy tremendously)

Home. In some ways this is the most difficult area of all to work on because our relations with our spouses, our children and ourselves are very much based on upbringing. We tend to internalize the behavior and beliefs of our own families. We receive these messages very early in life and they are as much a part of us as our arms and legs.

A real conflict occurs when what we would like to have as an adult differs from what we have been taught to have. You may want a satisfying sexual relationship but if your parents didn't have one or taught you that it was to be feared, you may set up your environment so that it doesn't occur. You may fight with your spouse to avoid intimacy, or you may pick a spouse who is not interested in sex. These are just a few of the hundreds of ways that people unconsciously set themselves up for frustration and stress.

If you are extremely uncomfortable with the personal life that you've constructed for yourself, you may need to work with a counselor. On a day-to-day level, however, there are certainly things that you can do to improve your life. Reading psychology books and inspirational texts, listening to tapes and repeating affirmations to replace the negative parental messages that you learned as a child can all help. Your belief system can slowly be programmed toward what will make you happy.

When I question patients, many of them seem to recognize what their problems are even if they aren't sure how to solve them. Many people communicate in a way that doesn't work. They either don't state their wishes directly, they do so in an aggressive and combative way, or they communicate as a victim about to be kicked.

If you know that you have a problem area, it might help to:

- Ask for feedback from the people around you. Ask your spouse or friends. Be open to the feedback. Don't "kill the messenger" by becoming angry or defensive.

- Negotiate your differences. Businesses collapse when bosses and employees don't listen to each other. Your home is no different. You would never think of screaming at your boss unless you wanted to be fired. Why scream at your children or friends? All it does is drain your energy. Bad communication habits cause stress, disrupt your autonomic nervous system, and can be an environmental trigger for PMS.

- It is necessary to sit down with other people and discuss problems in a way that can bring a positive result. Discussions work when two people give a little and take a little. This way everyone wins.

We would all like to have exactly what we want 100 percent of the time, but that doesn't happen in real life. For example, you may want to go out and socialize at parties on the weekends. Your spouse may want to stay home and watch TV.

The following way of expressing yourself will **NOT** work:

You (angry tone of voice): "It's all your fault. You keep me from having any fun. All we ever do is stay at home."

Even if you honestly feel this way, expressing it in an angry way will only bring an angry response. You won't be listened to. You may have better luck with:

You (concerned tone of voice): "I'm not happy with our social life. I would like to go out more often and you like to stay at home. How can we work out this problem?"

This can succeed only if you have a mate or friends who are open to discussing matters with you. But at least you will be part of the solution, not part of the problem.

Techniques for Relaxation

Many people think of relaxation as what we do while we are asleep. We Westerners tend to be very goal-oriented. We hurry through the day trying to complete tasks as fast as possible and then go on to the next ones. There is a continual sense of urgency—"I've got to get it done"—without much regard for how we get there. This tends to speed up the autonomic nervous system responses that lead to stress and tension and can worsen PMS. With the use of relaxation techniques, tasks get done in the same amount of time and the journey is much more enjoyable.

For example, as I write this book I set daily production goals for myself. To meet these goals I can either rush to get the work done as fast as I can or I can work in a leisurely way. When I work in a rushed manner, I become more nervous and tired by the end of the day. My back muscles feel sore from bending over the typewriter.

If I work in a leisurely way, I get out of my chair every hour to two and take a break. I stretch my cramped muscles, do some deep breathing exercises, and clear my mind. The surprise is that I get more work done the second way—and feel a lot more relaxed and energetic by the end of the workday.

For the last few years I have been teaching these relaxation methods to patients. We go over these exercises at my office or they learn them on their own using books and tapes that I suggest. Almost without exception they come back very enthusiastic about the results. They say that these exercises calm their minds and their bodies. They usually feel happier and more positive about their lives. They also note improvements in their physical health. A calm mind seems to calm the body: the autonomic nervous system slows down and the body chemistry normalizes.

Here are some simple exercises that I have found to be very helpful for women with PMS:

First Step. Find a comfortable position. For many women, this means lying on their backs. You may also to the exercises sitting up. Try to keep your spine as straight as possible. Your arms and legs should be uncrossed. It is important that your clothes be loose and comfortable.

Second Step. Focus your attention upon the exercises so that distracting thoughts do not interfere with your concentration. Close your eyes and take a few deep breaths, in and out. This will help to remove your thoughts from the problems and tasks of the day and begin to quiet your mind.

Exercise 1: Concentration

Look at a watch with a secondhand. Focus all of your attention upon the hands of the watch. For fifteen seconds don't let any other thoughts enter your mind. At the end of this time, notice your breathing. You will probably find that it has slowed down and is calmer. You may also feel less nervous.

Exercise 2: Deep Abdominal Breathing

Lie flat on your back with your knees pulled up. Keep your feet slightly apart. Try to breathe in and out through your nose.

Inhale deeply. As you breathe in allow your stomach to relax so that the air flows into your abdomen. Your stomach should balloon out as you breathe in. Visualize the lowest part of your lungs filling up with air. Imagine that the air you are breathing is filling your body with energy.

Exhale deeply. As you breathe out, imagine the air being pushed out from the bottom of your lungs to the top, as if a tube of toothpaste were being rolled up. As you exhale, imagine that you are sending love and peace with every breath.

Repeat this sequence until your breathing is slow and regular. Your entire body will feel relaxed. This breathing exercise will also strengthen muscles in your abdomen and chest. It is also very useful for anyone with respiratory problems.

Exercise 3: Discovering Muscle Tension

Lie in a comfortable position. Allow your right arm to rest limply, palm down, on the surface next to you.

Now raise just the hand, not the entire arm, and hold it there for fifteen seconds.

How does the top of your forearm feel? Does it feel tight and tense?

Now let your arm drop down and relax. The arm muscles will relax too. They should feel comfortable again.

As you lie there, notice any other parts of your body that carry tension. They will feel tight and a little sore. You may notice a constant dull aching. Tense muscles block blood flow and cut off the supply of nutrients to the tissues. The muscle is poorly oxygenated and in response produces lactic acid.

Exercise 4: Progressive Muscle Relaxation

Lie in a comfortable position. Allow your arms to rest limply, palms down, on the surface next to you. Practice your deep breathing from Exercise 2 as you do this exercise.

Clench your hands into fists and hold them tightly for fifteen seconds. As you do this, relax the rest of your body. Then let your hands relax.

Now tense and relax the following parts of your body in this order: your face, shoulders, back, stomach, pelvis, legs, feet, and toes. Hold each part tensed for fifteen seconds and then relax your body for thirty seconds before going to the next part.

Visualize the tense part contracting, becoming tighter and tighter. On relaxing, see the energy flowing into the entire body like a gentle wave, making all the muscles soft and pliable.

Finish the exercise by shaking your hands and imagining the remaining tension flowing out your fingertips.

This is a particularly useful exercise to do when you feel tension building up during the premenstrual period. It helps to discharge stress in a beneficial way.

Exercise 5: Meditation

Lie or sit in a very comfortable position.

Close your eyes and breathe deeply. Let your breathing be slow and relaxed.

Focus all of your attention on your breathing. Notice the movements of your chest and abdomen in and out.

Block out all other thoughts, feelings, and sensations. If you feel your attention wandering, bring it back to your breathing.

Say the word IN as you inhale. Say the word OUT as your exhale. Draw out the pronunciation of the word so that it lasts for the entire breath. The word IN sounds like this: i-i-i-i-n-n-n-n-n. The word OUT sounds like this: Ow-ow-w-w-w-w-t-t-t-t-t. Repeating these two words will help you to concentrate.

Do this exercise for as long as you are able to, up to several minutes.

This meditation requires you to sit quietly and engage in simple and repetitive activity. (This can be very difficult at first.) By emptying your mind you give yourself a rest. The metabolism of your body slows down. The brain wave slows from the fast beta wave that predominates during our normal working day to a slower alpha or theta wave. This slower pattern is what appears during sleep or in the period of deep relaxation just prior to falling asleep.

Meditating gives your mind a vacation from tension and worry. It is useful to do during the premenstrual period when every little stress is magnified into a monster. After meditating you may wonder what all your upset was about. You will see that situations are not as bad as you believed them to be.

Exercise 6: Affirmations

Sit in a comfortable position. Repeat the following affirmations. Repeat those that are particularly important to you three times.

- My body is strong and healthy.
- My female system is strong and healthy.
- My hormones are balanced and normal.
- My estrogen and progesterone levels are perfectly regulated.
- My body chemistry is balanced and normal.
- I go through my monthly menstrual cycle with ease and comfort.
- I barely know that my body is getting ready to menstruate.
- I feel wonderful each month before I menstruate.
- My mood is calm and relaxed throughout the month.
- I handle stress easily and competently.
- I desire a well-balanced and healthful diet.
- I enjoy eating delicious and nutritious food.
- My body wants food that is high in vitamins and minerals.
- I take time each day to relax and enjoy myself.
- I practice the relaxation methods that I enjoy.

During the time of the month when you are free of premenstrual symptoms, use these affirmations several times a day.

Your state of health is determined by the interaction between your mind and body. It is determined by the thousands of mental messages you send yourself each day with your thoughts. For example, if you do not like yourself, you will be constantly criticizing yourself: the way you look, talk, and act. This will be reflected in your body. Your shoulders will probably slump and your countenance will be lackluster and depressed.

When your body believes that it is sick, it behaves as if it were sick. That is part of the reason that you experience discomfort before your menstrual period. It is not enough to change your nutritional and exercise habits. You also need to change your belief system and the way in which you see your body. This technique of imaging your body the way you want it to be has been used to great benefit for patients with many types of disease.

In his book *Getting Well Again*, Carl Simonton, a cancer radiation therapist, used this technique with his patients. He asked them to imagine that they had strong immune systems capable of fighting a small, puny cancer (instead of the other way around). In a substantial number of cases he saw patients with very serious diseases go into remission.

Exercise 7: Visualizations

Close your eyes. Begin to breathe deeply. Inhale and let this air out slowly. Feel your body begin to relax.

Imagine that the premenstrual period is beginning and to your surprise you feel wonderful. Let a smile come on your face right now and see how good it feels. Let yourself feel happy for a few seconds.

Imagine yourself looking in a mirror. Actually see your body in your mind's eye. You are undressed or wearing a slip or shorts.

You look at your breasts and touch them. To your surprise they feel perfectly normal. They are not tender or swollen.

Look at your abdomen. See it flat and smooth. No bloating has accumulated this month.

Look at your face. It is smooth and relaxed. The smile is still on your face. You feel in command of yourself. You do not feel anxious, irritable, or depressed. Your mood is wonderful. As you look at yourself in the mirror, you know that you can handle any problems that come along, competently and with great ease.

Your complexion is clear and smooth. Touch your face and enjoy how nice it is to have clear skin in the time before your period.

Look at your entire body and enjoy the feeling of energy and optimism that is running through you. You have become very calm.

Now stop visualizing the scene and go back to deep breathing. You open your eyes and feel very good.

Visualizing this scene should take about forty-five seconds to one minute, perhaps longer if you choose to linger with a particular image. A visualization is successful when it allows you to actually change your feelings about a particular situation. Your visualization should begin to lay down the mental blueprint for a healthier body and more positive believe system about your health.

Hot Soak

This is an excellent method to induce relaxation. You can make a mineral bath that is similar to the mineral baths at health spas. Just run a hot tub of water and add one cup of sea salt and one cup of bicarbonate of soda. This is a highly alkaline mixture. It should be used only two or three times during the premenstrual period. It relieves menstrual cramps and helps calm premenstrual anxiety and irritability.

Soak for twenty minutes. You will probably feel very relaxed and sleepy after this bath. It is best taken just before going to sleep at night. Chances are you will sleep very well. You may wake up feeling refreshed and full of energy the next day.

Making the Improvement Permanent

Your state of health is deeply affected by your beliefs. When set in a positive manner, your mind can help to correct imbalances in your hormones and physiology. This chapter has introduced you to many different ways to reset your mind and body. Which exercises you practice will be a matter of your individual taste.

Try each one of them at least once. Experiment with them until you find the combination that works for you. Doing all seven will take no longer than fifteen minutes to a half hour, depending on how much time you wish to spend on each one.

Ideally the exercises should be done on a daily basis for at least a few minutes a day. Over time, they will help you to gain insight into your negative beliefs and change them into positive new ones. Your ability to cope with stress should be tremendously improved.

12

Exercise for PMS

When I was a teenager, exercise was never mentioned as a possible treatment for PMS. I was told only about aspirin, hot water bottles, and bed, none of which was effective. When my menstrual cramps would occur, I would go to bed and simply brave out the pain, hoping that it wouldn't last too long. I wish that I had known about the benefits of a well-conditioned body. I didn't find that out until I was in my internship year and began to swim and bicycle more as my period drew near. Since that time I've also noted the beneficial effects of exercise in many of my patients.

There are several physiological reasons why exercise relieves PMS. Premenstrual pain causes the breathing to become rapid and shallow. Women also tend to contract their muscles involuntarily when they are in pain or anticipate pain. Both shallow breathing and tight muscles can decrease the amount of blood flow and oxygenation to the tissues. This worsens the congestive symptoms of PMS greatly.

Aching in the ankles, feet, and pelvis is often due to fluid retention. (Some women notice visible swelling in their lower extremities premenstrually.) Exercise corrects all these conditions. The vigorous pumping action of the muscles that occurs with tennis, walking, swimming, and other activities moves blood and other fluids from the congestive organs. (Sexual intercourse and orgasm can make you feel better for the same reason.)

Exercise can prevent lower back pain and cramps by strengthening the back and abdominal muscles. Women who exercise regularly often report that their periods are shorter and that they bleed less.

There are also important psychological benefits to exercise. It reduces premenstrual anxiety and irritability by helping to balance the autonomic nervous system. It gives an effective way to discharge the overactive "fight or flight" pattern that many women experience. Most women note a deep sense of relaxation and peace after they exercise. This may be due to an increased output of endorphins (chemicals made by the brain that have a natural opiate effect and are thought to be the reason for the "runner's high" that many marathoners experience).

The benefits of aerobic exercise on PMS were reported in a study in the *Journal Psychosomatic Research*. This study compared 97 women who exercised on a regular basis to a group of 159 women with a sedentary lifestyle. The women who exercised regularly had much better concentration and fewer behavioral, mood, and pain symptoms during the premenstrual period than the women who did not exercise.

While moderate and frequent physical activity is beneficial, be aware that a vigorous program of exercise may cause menstrual irregularity. Young women who train for sports competitively or whose careers demand vigorous physical activity often experience a delay in the onset of their menstrual periods. By the age of 18, ten percent of ballet dancers are not yet menstruating. Women with normal cycles sometimes menstruate less often or stop entirely if they exercise vigorously.

Several reasons have been postulated for this. Ideally, the normal woman has about 22 percent body fat. The athletic woman may have as little as 10 percent. Since estrogen is synthesized by the fatty tissue as well as the ovaries, this can decrease the amount of circulating estrogen. Competitive training can also be emotionally very stressful. It can disrupt the menstrual cycle at the level of the hypothalamus, a part of the brain responsible for triggering the output of pituitary hormones. Many women athletes' cycles resume when their exercise level drops.

Certain types of exercise seem to be better than others for PMS. Walking at a fast pace in fresh air can be particularly beneficial. Try to walk in the early morning sunlight to increase your levels of natural vitamin D. Swimming is excellent for all-around toning and for cardiovascular health. Other enjoyable sports include bicycling, tennis, and moderate jogging.

Try to exercise as often as you can. Some form of exercise every day is preferable for general health. It is very important to increase the level of your activity for a week or two before the onset of your period. Try to exercise before your symptoms start. Don't wait until they reach crisis proportions.

13

Acupressure Massage

Western medicine sees the human body as a series of mechanical and chemical reactions. For example, the heart can fail mechanically as a pump. It can also fail chemically when essential minerals such as calcium and potassium are present in abnormal amounts.

Traditional Chinese Medicine has traditionally looked at the body in a different way. It is based on the belief that there exists a life energy or "biofield." This life energy is called chi. It is different yet similar to electromagnetic energy. Health is thought to occur when the chi is equally distributed throughout the body and is present in sufficient amounts. It is thought to energize all the cells and tissues of the body.

This life energy is thought to be distributed throughout the body in channels called meridians. This distribution system is analogous to blood and lymph vessels except that the latter distribute fluid and the meridians distribute a subtle energy. Meridians move energy through the body like invisible rivers. They flow deep into the interior of the body through the organ systems and at times surface on the skin. The place where the energy surfaces on the skin is called the acupuncture point. The electrical resistance of the skin at these points is slightly different from that of the surrounding skin.

Disease is thought to occur when the energy flow through a meridian stops or is blocked, then the corresponding internal organ system shows symptoms of disease. The meridian flow can be corrected by stimulating the points on the surface of the skin. These points can be treated either by hand massage, insertion of needles or electrical stimulus. When the normal flow of energy through the body is resumed, the body is believed to heal itself spontaneously.

Stimulation of the acupuncture points can be used to help relieve PMS. The simplest and most effective way is to use finger pressure. This can be done by you or a friend following simple instructions. It is safe and painless and does not require the use of needles. It can be used without the specialized years of training needed for insertion of needles.

I have used acupressure on my patients in my practice for many problems including pneumonia, viral infections, headaches, and muscles strains, as well as PMS. I have seen acupressure work on stubborn and resistant cases where nothing else seemed to be effective.

How to Perform Acupressure

1. Acupressure should be done either on yourself or by a friend when you are relaxed. Your room should be warm and quiet. Hands should be cleaned and nails trimmed to avoid bruising yourself. If your hands are cold, put them under warm water.

2. Choose the side of the body to work on that has the most discomfort (for example, your menstrual cramps may be worse on one side). If both sides are equally uncomfortable, choose whichever one you want. Working on one side seems to relieve symptoms on both sides. There appears to be a transfer of energy or information from one side to the other.

3. Hold each point indicated in the exercise with a steady pressure for one to three minutes. Pressure should be applied slowly with the tips or balls of the fingers. It is best to place several fingers over the area of the point. If you feel resistance or tension in the area on which you are applying tension, you may want to push a little harder. However, if your hand starts to feel tense or tired, lighten the pressure a bit. Make sure that your hand is comfortable. The acupressure point may feel somewhat tender. This means that the energy pathway or meridian is blocked.

4. During the treatment, the tenderness in the point should slowly go away. You may also have a subjective feeling of energy radiating from this point into the body. Don't worry if you do not feel it; not everybody does. The main goal is relief from your PMS.

5. Breathe gently while doing each exercise.

6. The point that you are to hold is shown in the photographs accompanying the text. All of these points correspond to specific points on the acupressure meridians.

7. You may massage the points once a day or more during the time that you have symptoms. You may even want to begin massaging the pressure points a day or two before you anticipate symptoms.

Acupressure Exercises

Exercise 1: General Balancing of the Energy Pathways

This sequence of points balances the energy flow of the entire body and benefits all of the meridians. It is the most calming of all sequences because it works directly on the spine and the brain. It balances the entire nervous system. It is excellent in helping to relieve the anxiety, mood swings, and irritability that more than 80 percent of women with PMS seem to suffer.

It relieves headaches and is also useful in balancing the energy of the reproductive tract.

Sit upright on a chair. Hold each step for 1 to 3 minutes.

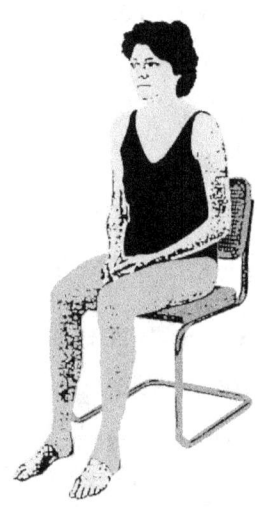

Left hand holds the point just below the base of the sternum. Right hand holds the point 2 inches below the navel.

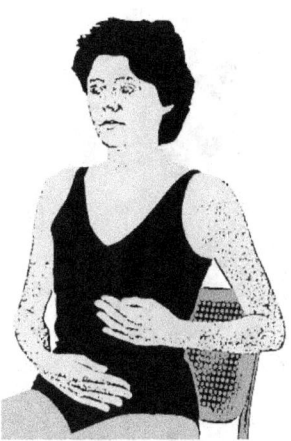

Left hand does not move. Right hand holds the point at the top of the pubic bone.

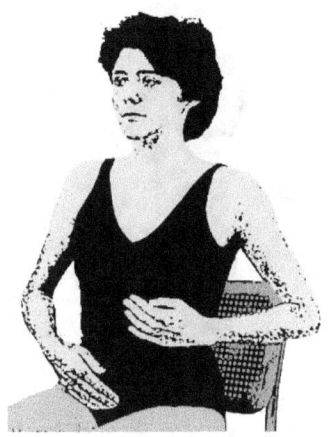

Left hand stays on the point just below the base of the sternum. Right hand holds the point at the bottom of the tailbone.

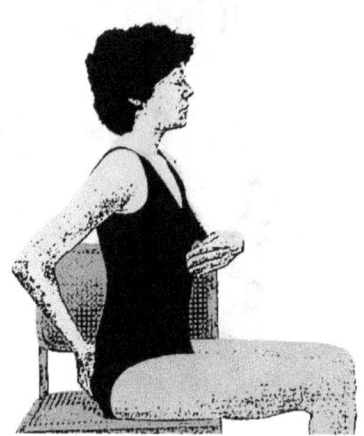

Left hand holds the point below the large vertebra (bone) at the base of the neck. Right hand is placed 1 inch above the waist on the spine.

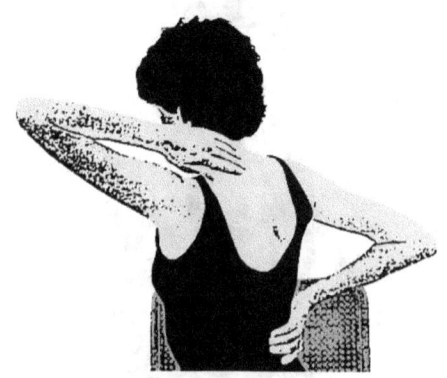

Left hand holds the point on the spine where it meets the base of the skull. Right hand stays 1 inch above the waist on the spine.

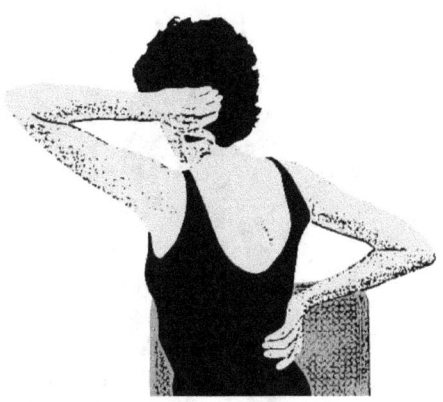

Left hand moves to the point between the eyebrows. Right hand holds the point on the top of the head.

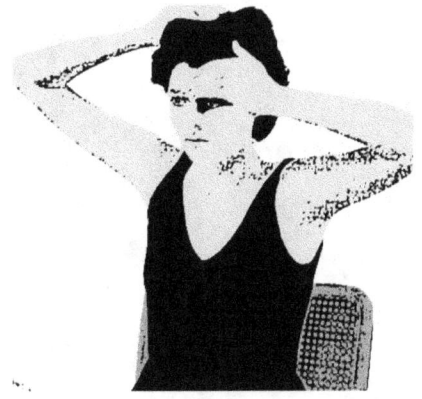

Left hand holds point between the nipples on the sternum. Right hand remains at the point on top of the head.

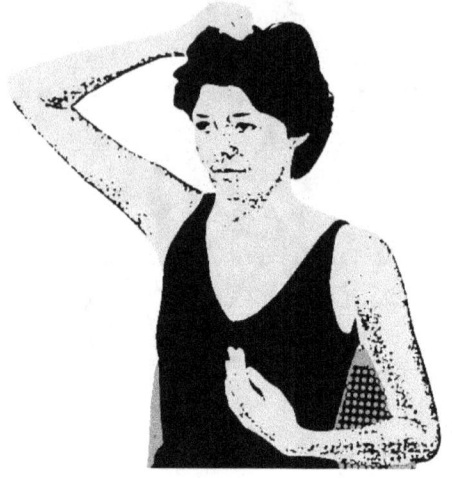

Exercise 2: Balances the Entire Reproductive System

This exercise alleviates all menstrual complaints, balances the energy of the female reproductive tract, and relieves low back pain and abdominal discomfort.

Equipment: This exercise uses a knotted hand towel to put pressure on hard to reach areas of the back. Place the knotted towel on these points while your two hands are on other points. This increases your ability to unblock the energy pathways of your body.

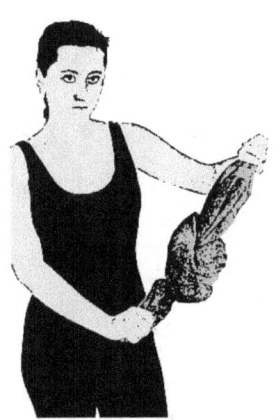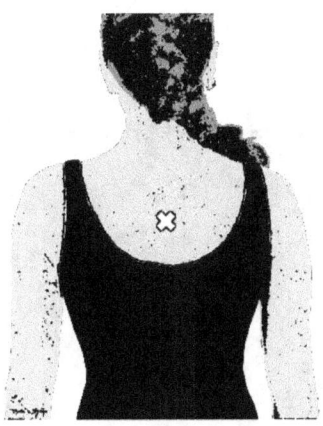

Lie on the floor with your knees up. As you lie down, place the towel between the shoulder blades on your spine. Hold each step 1 to 3 minutes.

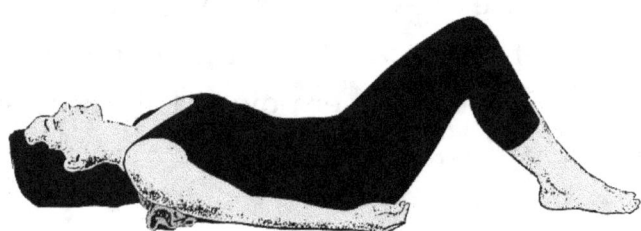

Cross your arms on your chest. Press your thumbs against the right and left inside upper arms.

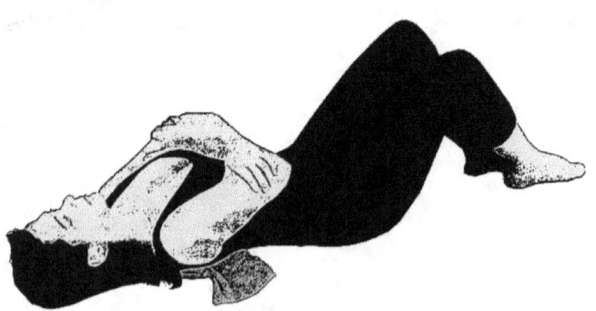

Left hand holds point at the base of the sternum (breastbone).

Right hand holds point at the base of the head (at the junction of the spine and the skull).

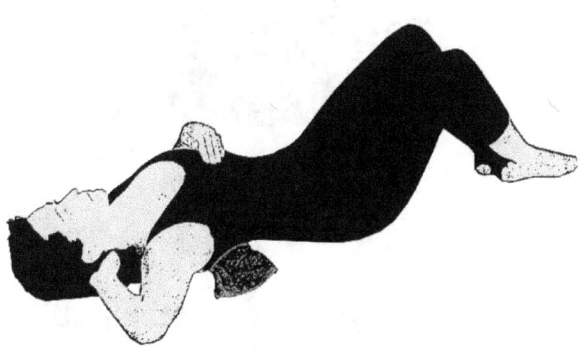

Interlace your fingers. Place them below your breasts. Fingertips should press directly against the body.

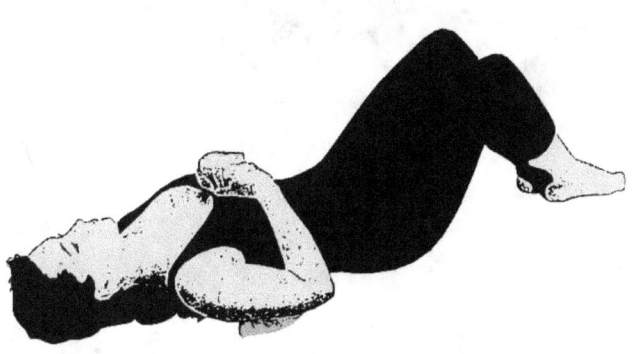

Move the knotted towel along the spine to the waistline.

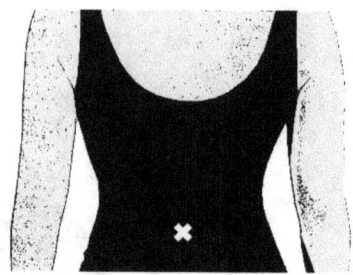

Left hand should be placed at the top of the pubic bone, pressing down.

Right hand holds point on tailbone.

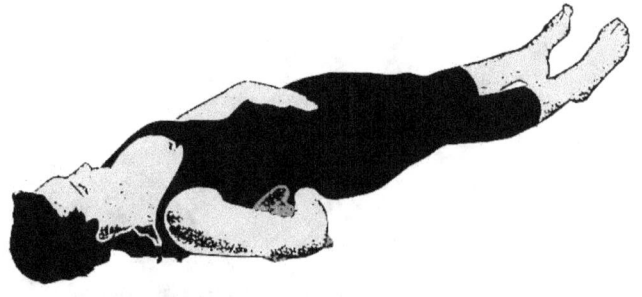

Exercise 3: Relieves Low Back Pain and Cramps

This exercise relieves menstrual cramps and low back pain by balancing points on the bladder meridian. It also balances the energy of the reproductive organs.

Sit on the floor and prop your back against a wall or a heavy piece of furniture. Hold each step for 1 to 3 minutes.

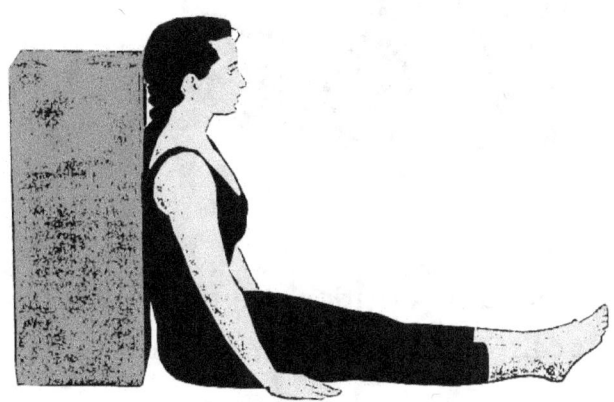

Alternative method: Lie on the floor and put your lower legs over the seat of a chair. Follow the exercise from that position.

Place left hand 1 inch above the waist on the muscle to the left side of the spine (muscle will feel firm and ropelike). Place right hand behind crease of the left knee.

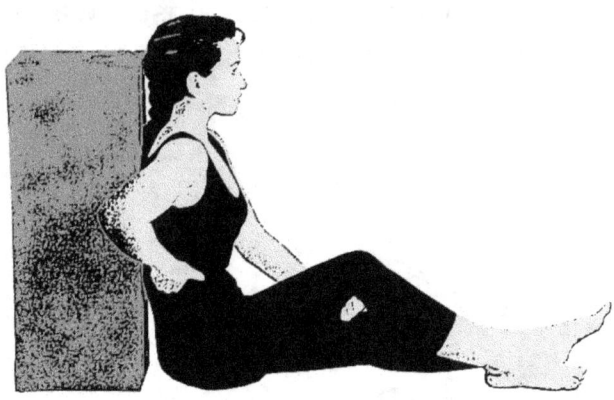

Left hand stays in the same position. Right hand is placed on the center of the back of the left calf. This is just below the fullest part of the calf.

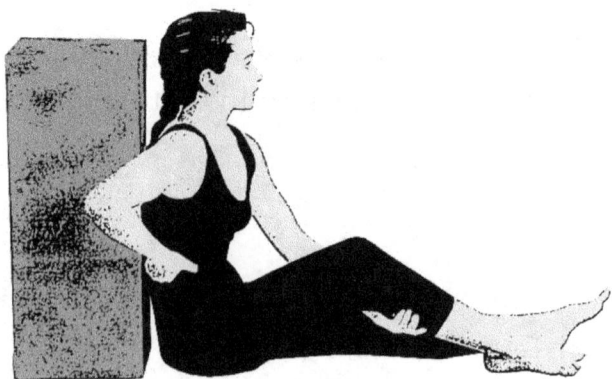

Left hand remains 1 inch above the waist on the muscle to the side of the spine. Right hand is placed just below the ankle bone on the outside of the left heel.

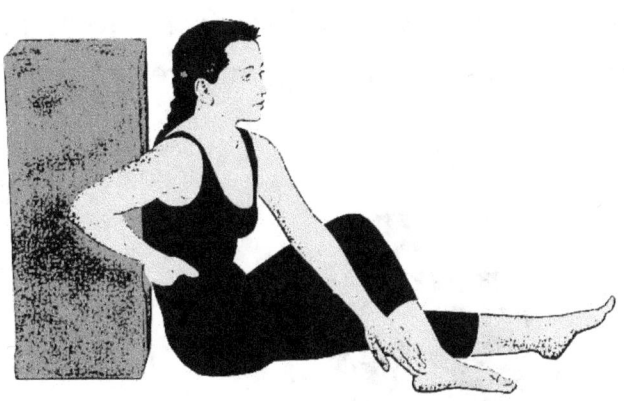

Left hand remains 1 inch above the waist on the muscle to the side of the spine. Right hand holds the front and back of the left little toe at the nail.

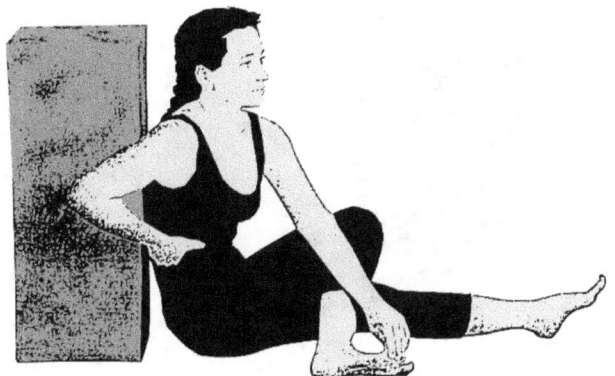

Exercise 4: Relieves Cramps, Bloating, Fluid Retention, Weight Gain

This sequence of points balances the energy flow of the spleen meridian. It is effective for relieving menstrual cramps. It relieves bloating and fluid retention and helps to minimize weight gain in the premenstrual period.

Sit up and prop your back against a chair, or lie down and put your lower legs on a chair. Hold each step for 1 to 3 minutes.

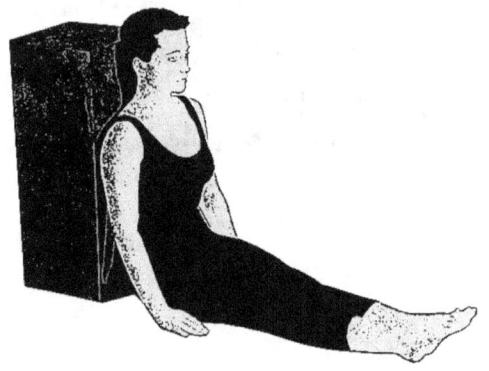

Left hand is placed in the crease of the groin where you bend your leg, one-third to one-half way between the hip bone and the outside edge of the pubic bone. Right hand holds a spot 2 to 3 inches above the knee.

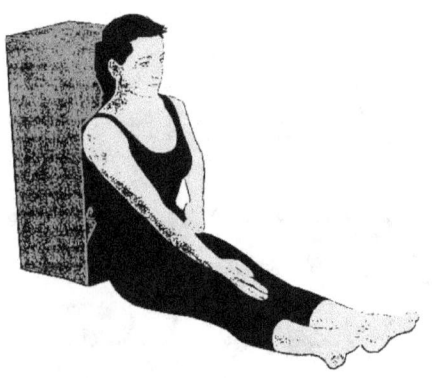

Left hand remains in the crease of the groin. Right hand holds point below inner part of knee. To find the point, follow the curve of the bone just below the knee. Hold the underside of the curve with your fingers.

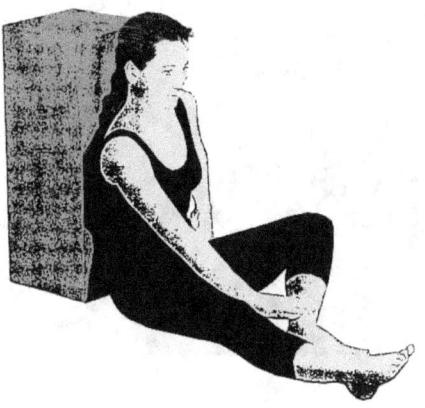

Left hand remains in the crease of the groin. Right hand holds the inside of the shin. To find this point, go four finger widths above the ankle bone. The point is just above the top finger.

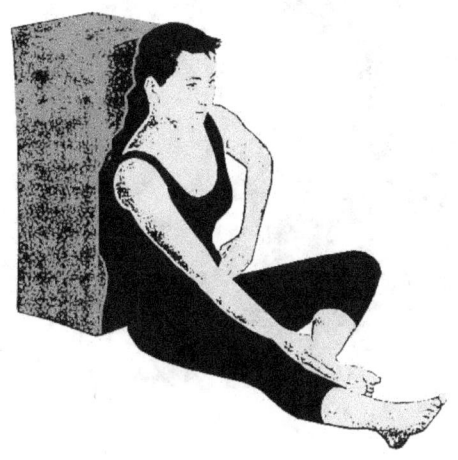

Left hand remains in the crease of the groin. Right hand holds the edge of the instep. To find the point, follow the big toe bone up until you hit a knobby, prominent small bone.

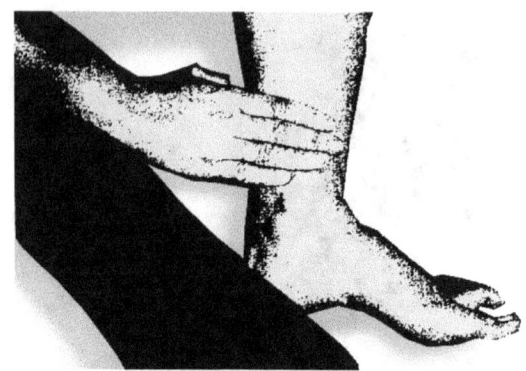

Left hand remains in the crease of the groin. Right hand holds the big toe over the nail, front and back of the toe.

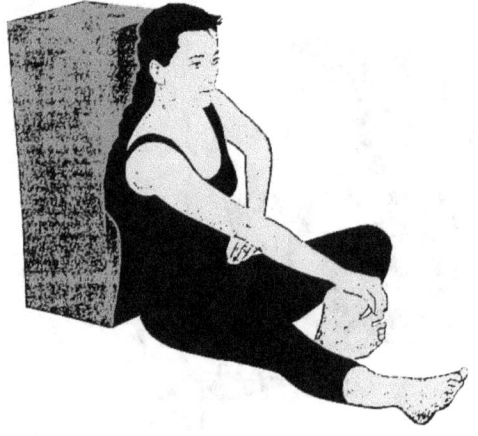

Exercise 5: Relieves Nausea

This exercise relieves premenstrual nausea. This usually occurs in conjunction with cramps and low back pain.

Lie on the floor or sit up. Hold these points 1 to 3 minutes.

Left index finger is placed in navel and pointed slightly toward the head. Right hand holds point at the base of the head.

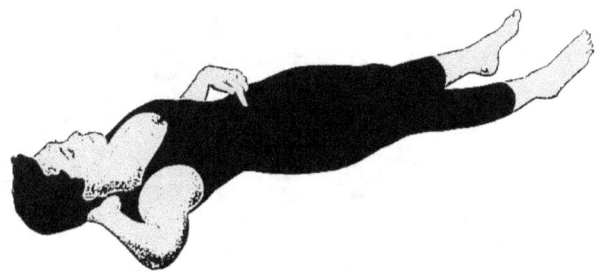

Exercise 6: Relieves Acne

This exercise relieves acne and helps to relieve hives.

Sit on the floor with the knees bent. Hold each step 1 to 3 minutes.

Left hand holds left calf. Right hand holds right calf.

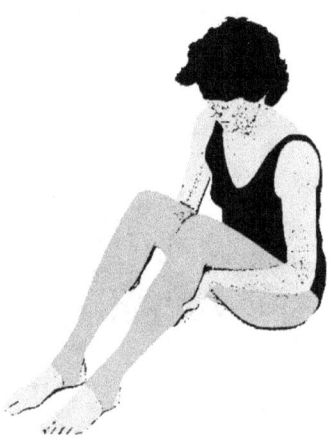

Cross arms. Left hand holds right calf. Right hand holds left calf.

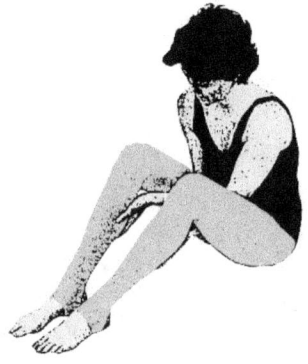

Exercise 7: *Relieves Depression, Headaches, Tightness of Neck and Shoulders, and Hypoglycemia*

The neck and shoulders generally carry a great deal of tension. Tightness in this area can act as a bottleneck and impede the energy flow of the entire body. Thus the entire body is energized by this exercise. It also relieves depression.

A major treatment point for hypoglycemia is worked on in this exercise. This may help reduce the excessive cravings for sweets that some women notice before their periods.

Sit comfortably or lie down. Hold each step 1 to 3 minutes.

Left hand holds point at the top of the shoulder blade, 1 to 2 inches to the side of the spine. The point is between the shoulder blade and the spine. It may feel firm and resistant. Right hand holds the same point on the right side.

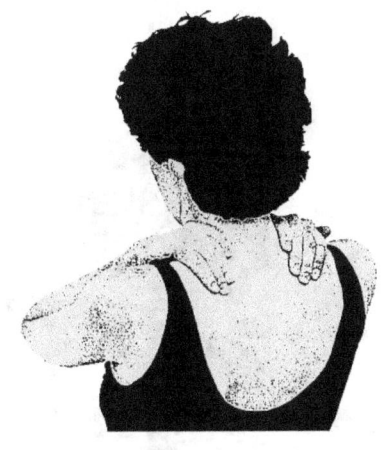

Left hand holds points slightly to the back of the top of the shoulder where the neck meets the shoulder. Right hand holds the same point on the right side.

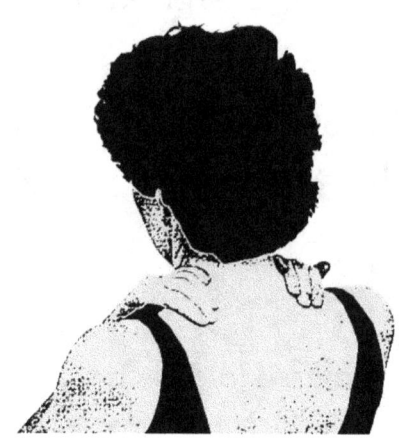

Left hand holds the point halfway up the neck, fingers sit on the muscle next to the spine. Right hand holds the same point on the right side.

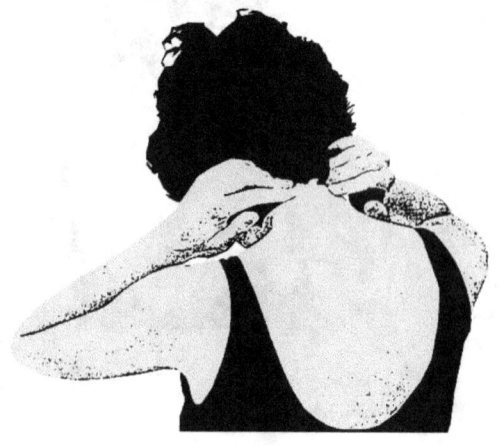

Left hand holds the point at the base of the skull 1 to 2 inches out from the spine. Right hand holds the same point on the right side.

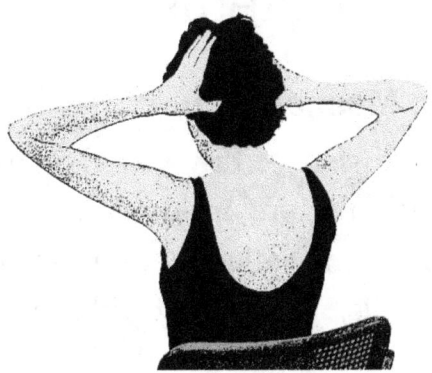

14

Massage of the Neurolymphatic and Neurovascular Systems

The Neurolymphatic Massage Points

The lymphatic system consists of tiny vessels that lead from the periphery of the body to the neck region. From there they empty into the veins leading to the heart. The lymphatics act as a drainage system, gathering up waste products from cells, dead white blood cells, bacteria, and other debris. Once the debris is moved from the lymphatics to the bloodstream, it is processed and excreted from the body. The lymph fluid moves through its channels by mild contractions of the lymph ducts and the surrounding skeletal muscles.

If a person overburdens the lymph system by eating improperly or not exercising, lymphatic fluid can accumulate and cause congestion in a particular area of the body. This was first noted by Dr. Frank Chapman, an osteopath who practiced in the early part of this century. He found that when the energy flow to the lymphatic system is blocked, reflex points regulating the flow of lymph turn off, shutting down the overburdened system like circuit breakers. These reflex points are located primarily on the back and chest. They are small and grainy in texture, usually no larger than a pea, and can be felt over a muscle group. When there are blocks, pain and congestion appear in that area. Chapman found that this correlated to organ-system and endocrine dysfunction. Firm rubbing of these points can decrease the symptoms significantly.

You may want to try massaging these points, especially if the acupressure points do not work. If lymphatic congestion is the cause, pain should decrease over a few days. Locate the points on your body as indicated by the following photographs. Massage deeply and firmly with the fingers for twenty to thirty seconds.

Neurolymphatic Point 1: Relieves Anxiety, Mood Swings, Irritability, Depression, Breast Tenderness, and Bloating

Massage each area shown in the photographs for 20 to 30 seconds.

Front of the body: Area is located between the fifth and sixth ribs, extending from the nipple to the breastbone on the right and left sides.

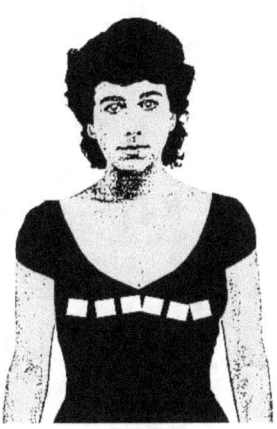

Back of the body: Area is located one inch to either side of the spine (at the levels of the fifth, sixth, and seventh vertebrae). Look for the soft area between the bones and then move 1 inch to the side.

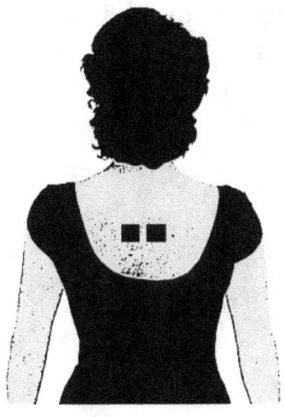

Neurolymphatic Point 2: Relieves Fluid Retention, Weight Gain, and Acne

Massage each area shown in the photographs for 20 to 30 seconds.

Front of the body: Area is located 1 inch up from the navel, 1 inch to either side.

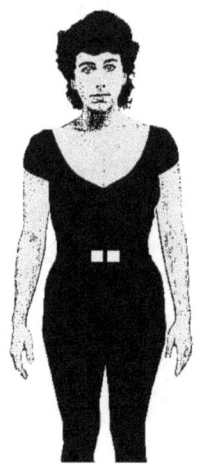 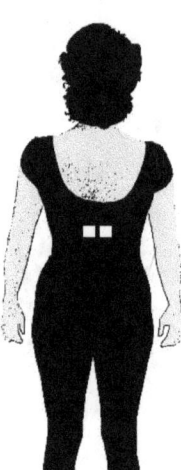

Back of the body: Area is located 1 inch to either side of the spine (between the twelfth thoracic and the first lumbar vertebrae). This is just below the level of the last ribs.

Neurolymphatic Point 3: Use for Carbohydrate Craving, Dizziness, Fatigue

Massage each area shown in the photographs for 20 to 30 seconds.

Front of the body: Area is located 2 inches above the navel and 1 inch to either side.

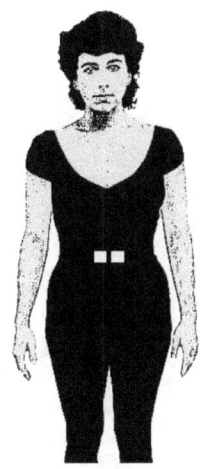 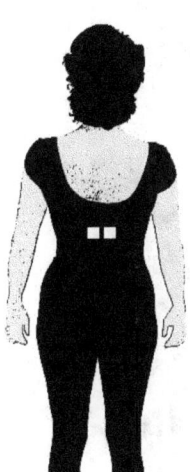

Back of the body: Area is located 1 inch to either side of the spine at the level of the last ribs. (This is between the tenth and eleventh thoracic vertebrae and the eleventh and twelfth thoracic vertebrae.)

Neurolymphatic Point 4: Use for Carbohydrate Craving, Dizziness, Fatigue

Massage each area shown in the photographs for 20 to 30 seconds.

Front of the body: On the left side of the chest between the seventh and eighth ribs, 1 to 2 inches to the side of the midline.

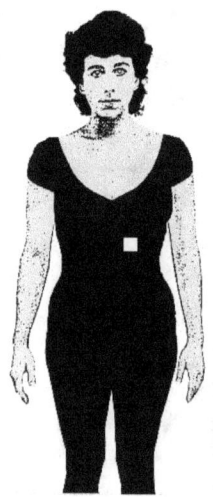 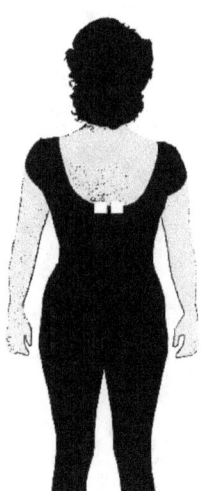

Back of the body: One inch to either side of the spine (between the seventh and eighth thoracic vertebrae).

Neurolymphatic Point 5: Relieves Cramps, Low Back Pain

Massage each area shown in the photographs for 20 to 30 seconds.

Front of the body: Points are located at the upper and inner edges of the pubic bone.

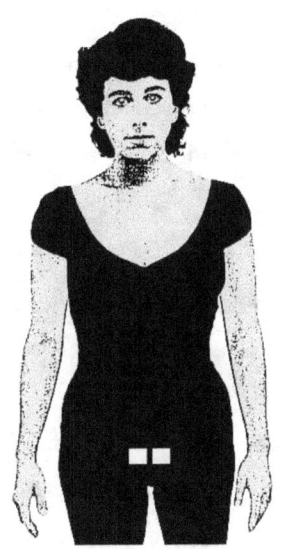 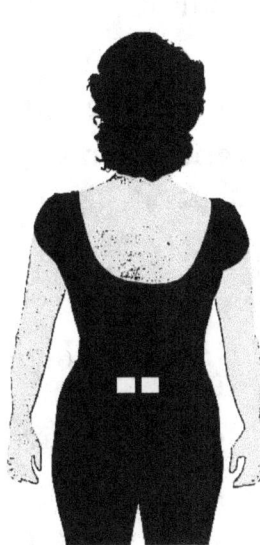

Back of the body: One inch to either side of the spine (at the upper edge of the second lumbar vertebra).

The Neurovascular Holding Points

The neurovascular holding points were discovered by Terrence Bennett, a pioneer in the field of chiropractic. He found that stimulating skin areas with light touch could improve blood circulation in deep organ systems. He observed these changes in many patients by watching their organs through a fluoroscope while pressure was being applied to their skin.

Neurovascular points are located mainly on the head. They should be touched lightly with the pads of the fingers. After holding the points for a few seconds, a slight pulsation will be felt. This pulse is not related to the heartbeat. It is thought to be the pulsation of the microcapillary bed in the skin. These points can be held from twenty seconds to five minutes, depending on the severity of the problem. For PMS, their greatest use is in treating symptoms related to emotional upset.

Neurovascular Point 1: Relieves Anxiety, Mood Swings, Irritability, Depression, and Tension Headaches

Points can be held for up to five minutes. Concentrate on what-ever feelings or situations are upsetting you. Try to feel your upset as strongly as you can. After a time, you will find that you have difficulty concentrating on the problem. It will seem to fade and you may feel much more peaceful at the end of the exercise. This is the most important exercise for relieving emotional upsets.

Frontal eminence: Located on the forehead between the eye-brows and the hairline.

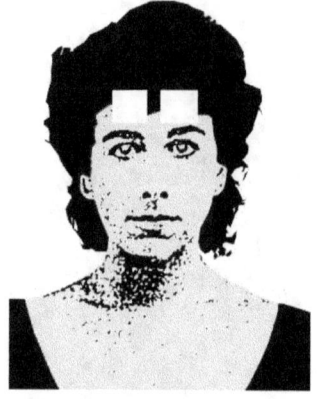

Neurovascular Point 2: Relieves Anxiety, Mood Swings, Irritability, Depression, and Fatigue

Point can be held up to five minutes. Hold until negative emotion fades and energy improves.

Parietal fontanel: Located at the back of the head in the midline. This corresponds to the soft spot on the back of a baby's head.

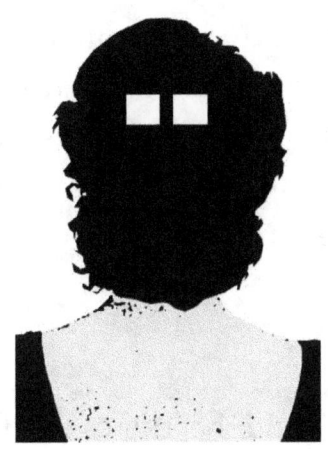

15

Stretches for PMS

I have chosen stretches for PMS that promote balance and harmony as well as helping to relieve PMS symptoms. Done properly, these exercises promote health on all levels — physical, mental, emotional, and spiritual.

It is important that you take a few minutes to focus and concentrate on these stretches before you actually do them. First your mind visualizes how the exercise is to look and then your body follows with the correct placement of the stretch. The exercises are done through slow, controlled stretching movements. This slowness allows you to have greater control over your body movements. You minimize the possibility of injury and maximize the benefit to the particular part of the body that your attention is being directed toward.

Warm Ups

The following exercises should be done the first week or two of your program. Warm-ups promote flexibility and mobility throughout the body. They will prepare you for the specific exercises you will be using to help correct PMS. Try each warm-up exercise at least once. Then put together your own routine. You may find that you want to do all six of them on a regular basis or perhaps only a few. Warm-ups should always precede the PMS corrective exercises.

How to Perform Stretches for PMS

1. These stretches should be performed in a relaxed and unhurried manner. Be sure to set aside adequate time, between ten to thirty minutes, so that you do not feel rushed. Your work area should be quiet, peaceful, and uncluttered.

2. Choose a flat area and work on a mat or a blanket. This will make you more comfortable while you do the exercises. Always rest for a few minutes after doing PMS stretches.

3. Wear loose, comfortable clothing. It is better that you work without socks to give your feet complete freedom of movement and to prevent slipping.

4. Wait at least two hours after eating to exercise. Evacuate your bowels or bladder before you begin the exercises.

5. Try to practice these movements on a regular basis. Every day for a few minutes is best, particularly when you have PMS. If that is not possible, then try to practice them every other day.

6. Pay close attention to the instructions when beginning an exercise. Look at the placement of the body as shown in the photographs. This is very important, for if the pose is practiced properly, you are much more likely to have relief of your PMS.

7. Try to visualize the pose in your mind, then follow with proper placement of the body.

8. Move slowly through the pose. This will help promote flexibility of the muscles and prevent injury.

9. Follow the breathing instructions in the exercise. Most important, do not hold your breath. Always allow your breathing to flow. It is important that you time your breathing with the placement of the body position.

10. Don't be discouraged if you can't do as much as the model in these illustrations.

Stretch 1

This exercise improves circulation to the upper half of the body and energizes and stimulates it. It also loosens and stretches tense muscles in the upper body, especially the shoulders and back, and expands the lungs.

Stand easily. Arms should be at your sides; feet are hip distance apart.

Bring your arms back slowly and gracefully until you can clasp them behind your back.

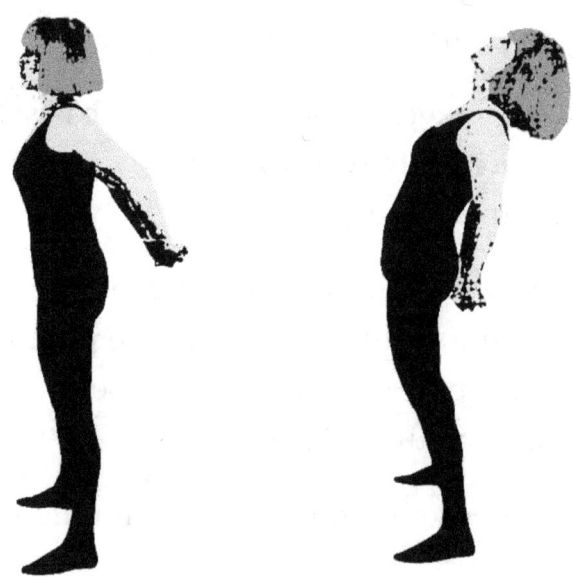

Exhale, then straighten your clasped hands and arms as far as you can without discomfort. Remember to stand upright; body should not bend forward. Breathe deeply into chest.

As you hold your breath, bend forward at the waist, bringing your clasped hands and arms up over your back.

Relax your neck muscles and keep your knees straight. Hold for a few seconds.

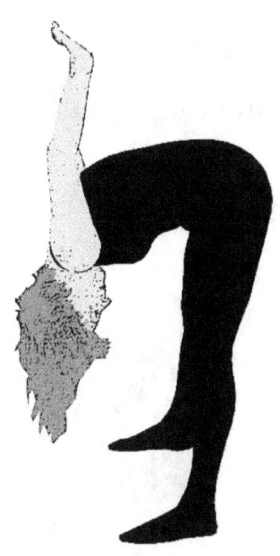

Exhale as you return to the upright position. Unclasp your hands and allow your arms to rest easily at your sides.

Repeat entire sequence 3 times.

Stretch 2

This exercise relieves tension in the hips and shoulders, strengthens the legs and back, and aids in balance.

Stand easily with your arms at your sides. Raise your right arm slowly overhead. Shift your weight to your right leg.

Catch your left ankle with your left hand, bending leg at the knee. You will be balancing yourself on your right leg.

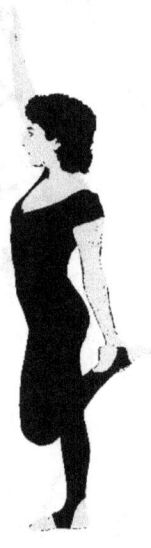

Gently stretch your back by bringing your right hand back a few inches and pulling your left leg up a few inches and moving it away from your body. This should be done slowly. The left arm remains straight to open the shoulder.

Slowly return to your original resting position. Repeat exercise on opposite foot.

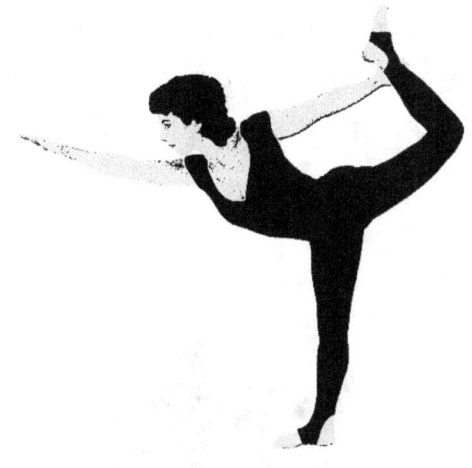

Stretch 3

This exercise relieves stiffness and tension in the neck, lubricates the vertebrae, and strengthens the muscles of the neck. You may want to repeat this exercise several times a day if your neck is particularly stiff. You may hear a gritty sound at first. This can accompany stiff and contracted muscles. Visualize your neck rolling slowly and smoothly on ball bearings as you do this exercise.

Sit in a chair with your arms and shoulders relaxed. First breathe in deeply, then exhale and allow your head to come all the way forward to your chest, keeping the spine straight. Hold for a few breaths.

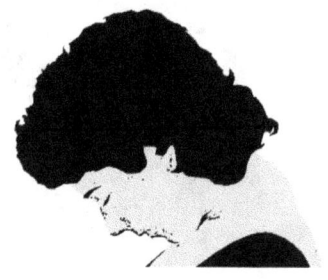

Exhale and bring your right ear to the right shoulder, keeping the right shoulder completely relaxed. Hold for a few breaths.

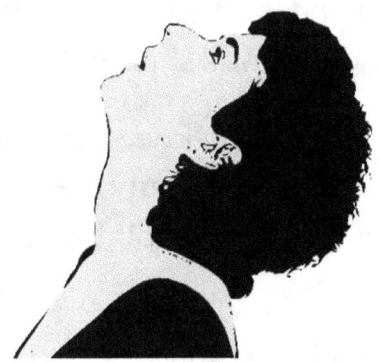

Exhale and allow your head to drop back, keeping the spine straight and the shoulders relaxed. Hold for a few breaths.

Bring your left ear to the left shoulder, keeping your left shoulder relaxed. Hold for a few breaths.

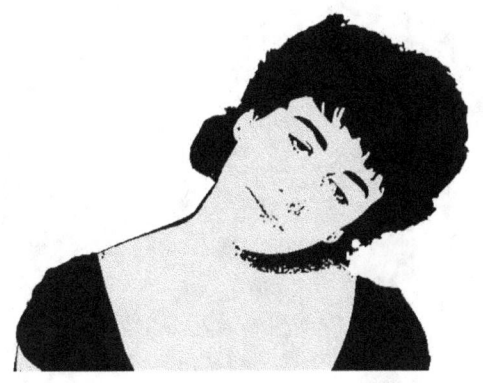

Bring your head to the original position, keeping your chin forward. Slowly repeat the exercise moving in the opposite direction.

Stretch 4

This exercise massages the entire neck and spine and flexes the vertebral column. It will invigorate and energize you, reducing fatigue.

Lie on your back. Bend and raise your knees to your chest, clasping them with your hands. Hands should be interlocked below knees.

Raise your head toward your knees and gently rock back and forth on your curved spine. Note the roundness of your back and shoulders. Keep the chin tucked in as you roll back. Avoid rolling back too far on your neck.

Rock back and forth 5 to 10 times.

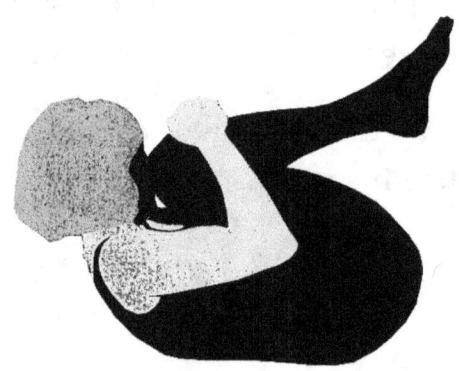

Stretch 5

This exercise strengthens the back and abdominal muscles, improves blood circulation through the pelvis, and calms anxiety and nervousness.

Lie down and press the small of your back into the floor. This permits you to use your abdominal muscles without straining your lower back.

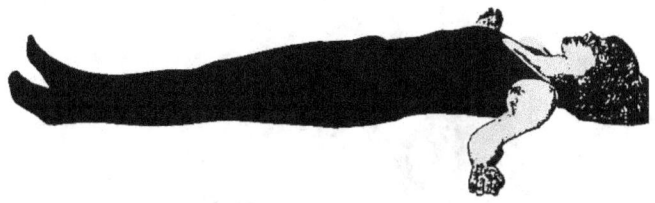

Raise your right leg slowly while breathing in. Keep your back flat on the floor and let the rest of your body remain relaxed. Move your leg very slowly; imagine your leg being pulled up smoothly by a spring. Do not move your leg in a jerking manner. Hold for a few breaths.

Lower your leg and breathe out. Repeat the same exercise on your left side. Then alternate legs, repeating the exercise 5 to 10 times.

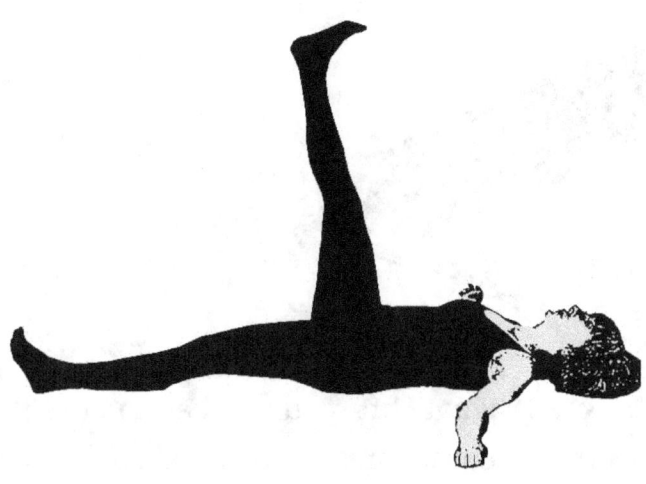

Stretch 6

This exercise emphasizes freer pelvic movement with controlled breathing, energizes and rejuvenates the female reproductive tract, and tones the abdominal organs (pancreas, liver, and adrenals). It may also help relieve premenstrual carbohydrate craving and dizziness. It may even help to relieve premenstrual acne.

Lie on your back with your knees bent and your feet on the floor close to your buttocks.

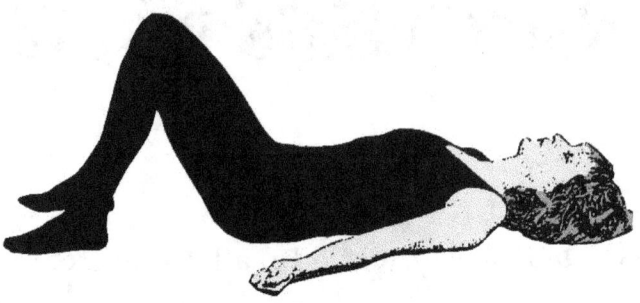

Exhale and press the lower back into the floor, raising the buttocks slightly. Arch the back slightly. Inhale and lift your lower back off the floor. This stretches the region from the sternum to the pelvis.

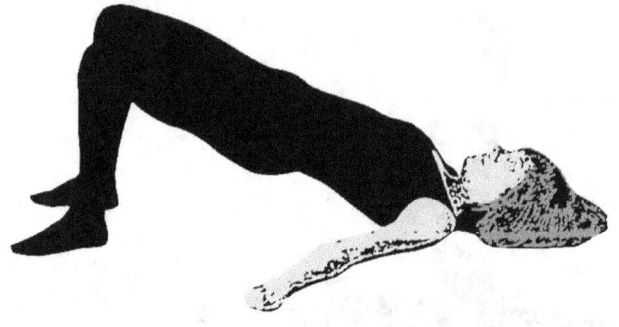

Repeat this exercise 10 times. Always lift your navel up on the in-breath. Always elongate your spine and press the lower back down on the out-breath.

Stretches for Relieving PMS

These exercises should be done after mastering the warm-ups. You may want to start these on week 2 of your program (or week 3 if you prefer to pace yourself a little slower). These exercises energize the entire female tract and relieve low back problems. They also relieve specific symptoms of PMS.

Stretch 7

This exercise relieves low back pain and strengthens the spine. It improves blood circulation to the pelvic region and encourages chest expansion and lung elasticity. It also elevates mood and can help to relieve depression.

Lie on your stomach with your chin on the floor and your feet together. Place your palms flat on the floor, underneath your shoulders.

As you inhale, lift your head up, stretching your neck back. Then, raise your chest, using your arms and back muscles.

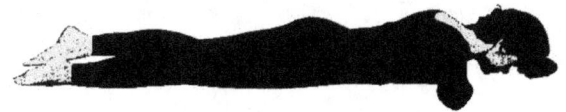

As you complete the inhalation, arch your body all the way up, keeping your hips on the ground.

As you hold this position, exhale deeply. Then, breathe deeply and slowly, inhaling and exhaling for 30 seconds.

Lower yourself part way, using your arms for support. Holding the body at this angle, breathe deeply for 30 seconds.

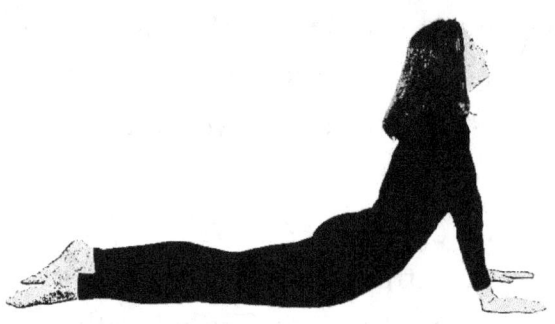

Then let your body come all the way down. Relax with your head turned to one side and your arms resting gently on the floor. Close your eyes and relax for several minutes.

Stretch 8

This exercise strengthens the lower back, abdomen, buttocks, and legs; and prevents low back pain and cramps. It helps to reduce weight in the thighs and hips and tighten and firm the skin in these areas. It also energizes the entire female reproductive tract, thyroid, liver, intestines, and kidneys.

Lie face down on the floor. Make fists with both your hands and place them under your hips. This prevents compression of the lumbar spine while doing the exercise.

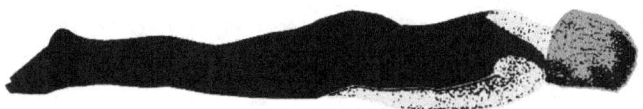

Straighten your body and raise your right leg with an upward thrust as high as you can, keeping your hips on your fists. Hold for 5 to 20 seconds if possible.

Lower the leg and slowly return to your original position. Repeat on the left side, then with both legs together. Remember to keep your hips resting on your fists. Repeat 10 times.

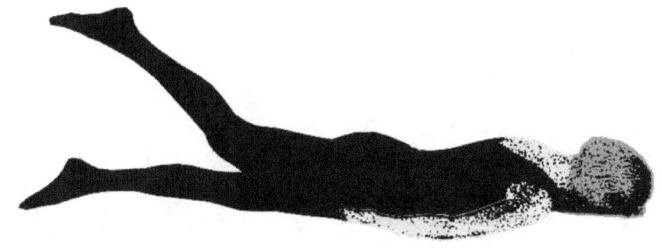

Stretch 9

This exercise stretches the entire spine and helps to relieve low back pain and cramps. It stretches the abdominal muscles and strengthens the back, hips, and thighs. It also stimulates digestive organs and endocrine glands. It may help to relieve sugar craving, oily skin, and acne. And finally, it relieves depression, fatigue, and lethargy, improving your energy and elevating your mood.

Lie face down on the floor, arms at your sides.

Slowly bend your legs at the knees and bring your feet up toward your buttocks.

Reach back with your arms and carefully take hold of first one foot and then the other. Flex your feet to make grasping them easier.

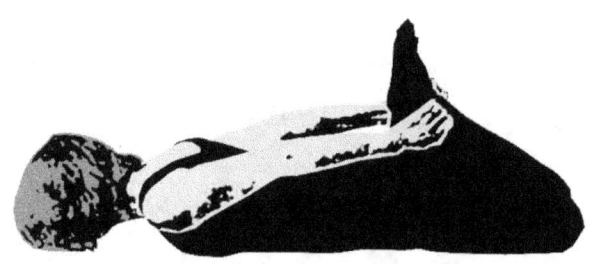

Inhale and raise your trunk from the floor as far as possible. Lift your head and elevate your knees off the floor.

Squeeze the buttocks. Imagine your body looking like a gently curved bow. Hold for 10 to 15 seconds.

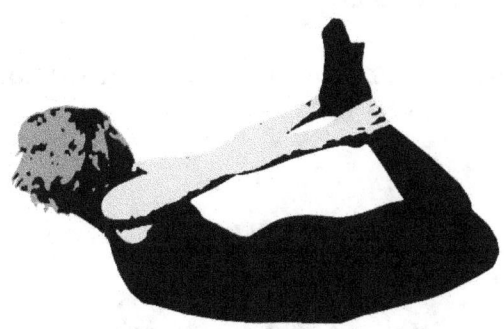

Slowly release the posture. Allow your chin to touch the floor and finally release your feet and return them slowly to the floor. Return to your original position. Repeat 5 times.

Stretch 10

This exercise gently stretches the lower back. It is excellent for calming anxiety and irritability. It also relieves menstrual cramps.

Sit on your heels. Bring your forehead to the floor, stretching the spine as far over your head as possible.

Close your eyes. Hold for as long as this is comfortable.

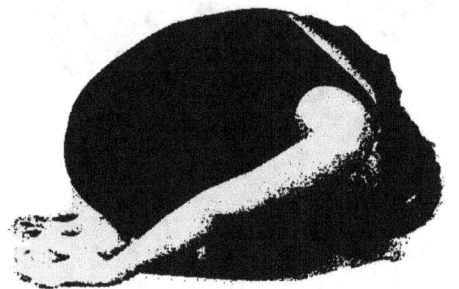

Stretch 11

This exercise opens the entire pelvic region, energizes the female reproductive tract, and relieves bloating and fluid retention in legs and feet.

Lie on your back with your legs against the wall and extended out in a V or an arc, and your arms extended to the sides.

Hips should be as close to the wall as possible, buttocks on the floor. Spread legs apart as far as you can while still remaining comfortable. Breathing easily, hold for 1 minute, allowing the inner thighs to relax.

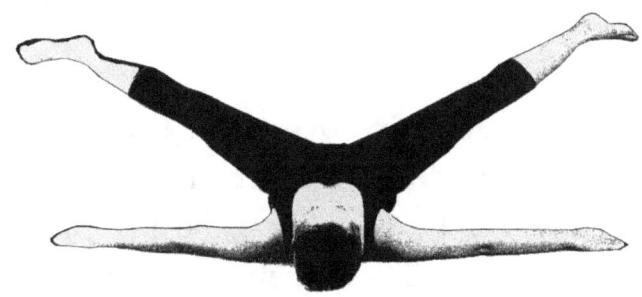

Bring legs together and hold for 1 minute.

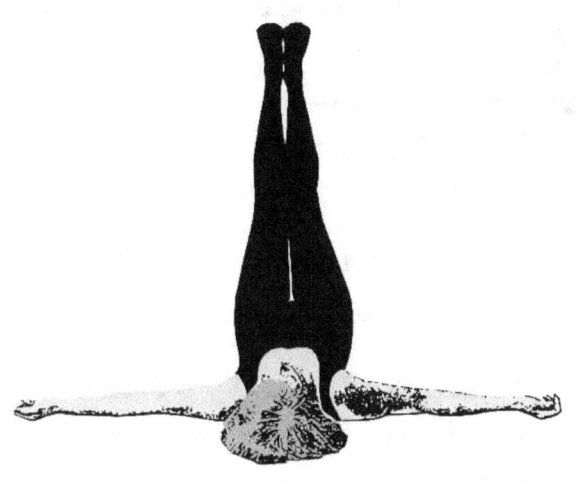

Stretch 12

This exercise improves the elasticity of the spine, strengthens the back and relaxes the abdomen and neck. It helps to reduce weight in the hips, thighs, legs, and abdomen. It improves circulation to the brain. It also reduces swelling and fluid retention in the legs and ankles.

Put a chair on your mat. Lie on your back, facing upward away from the chair. Arms are at your sides and palms are facing downward so that they press against the floor. Legs should be together.

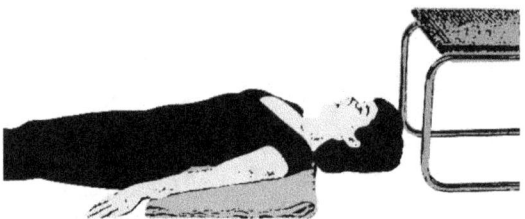

Slowly raise your legs and hips over your head until your toes touch the chair. This should be done without jerking, so bend your knees if necessary. Lift the spine by stretching the back muscles as much as possible. This exercise will alleviate compression of the lumbar spine.

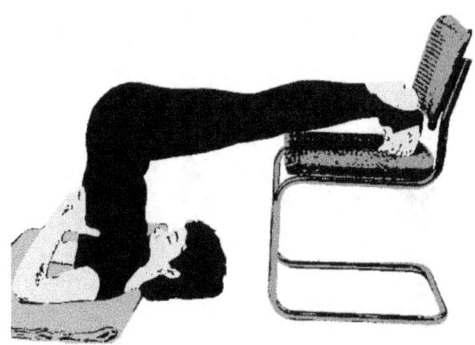

To come out of this posture, bend your knees and roll down slowly onto your back. Return to your original position.

(*This exercise is usually done by bringing the legs and hips over the head until the toes touch the floor, but bringing the feet all the way to the floor could be harmful for women with PMS, since they often have a concavity of the back.*)

Stretch 13

This exercise relieves anxiety and irritability and reduces eye tension and swelling of the face. It relieves menstrual cramps and low back pain if a rolled towel is placed under the knees.

Lie on your back with a rolled towel placed under your knees. Your arms should be at your sides, palms up.

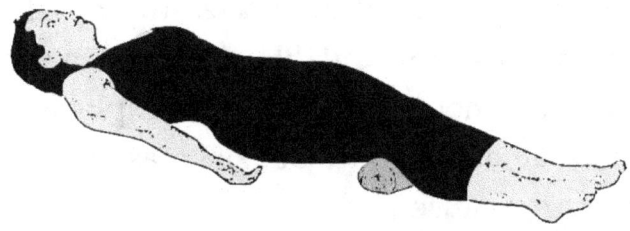

Close your eyes and relax your whole body. Inhale slowly, breathing from the diaphragm. As you inhale, visualize the energy in the air around you being drawn in through your entire body. Imagine that your body is porous and open like a sponge, so that this energy can be drawn in to revitalize every cell of your body.

Exhale slowly and deeply, allowing every ounce of tension to be drained from your body.

16

Treating PMS with Drugs

Drug treatment of PMS comes last in this book because this is a self-help book, but if your symptoms of PMS are severe, you may well want to go to your doctor first for the rapid symptomatic relief drugs can offer. Then, by following the self-help program, you should be able to cut back your dosage fairly quickly, and, unless you have a severe case, eventually give up the drug completely.

There have been some wonderful advances in the field of medicine and pharmacology. Treatments are available now for certain PMS symptoms, particularly cramps and mood swings, that simply were not around ten years ago. This is due in part to our increased awareness about the chemical imbalances that cause PMS.

Antiprostaglandin Medication

Particularly noteworthy are the medications that control menstrual cramps or primary dysmenorrhea. Primary dysmenorrhea refers to the types of cramps where no physical lesion is found to be causing the pain. (In contrast, secondary dysmenorrhea is due to lesions like fibroid tumors of the uterus or scarring due to pelvic inflammatory disease.)

Much research has been done to determine the cause of menstrual cramps. It is now known that it is caused by imbalances in prostaglandins. These are chemicals produced by the lining of the uterus. Their levels increase prior to menstruation. There are many types of prostaglandins that cause either relaxation or contraction of the uterus. The series-2 prostaglandins are primarily responsible for causing uterine contractions, in contrast to the series-1 prostaglandins which cause relaxation. If excess prostaglandin is produced or if there is an excess of series-2 over series-1, the uterus contracts too actively, causing cramping and pain.

Luckily, the cramp-causing prostaglandins can be suppressed. Drugs used in treating inflammatory diseases like arthritis were found to inhibit both prostaglandin synthesis and activity. These drugs include Indocin, Motrin, and Ponstel. These medications have been approved by the FDA for the treatment of menstrual pain and are being used widely today. Although these drugs are generally considered to be safe, they can have serious side effects and, like most drugs, require careful monitoring by doctor and patient.

Progesterone

Progesterone is one of the most commonly prescribed treatments for PMS today. Unlike the progesterone that women make in their own bodies in the corpus luteum of the ovary, the progesterone used in PMS treatment is primarily derived from soybean and wild yam sources. While recent research studies do not support the claim that PMS is due to a progesterone deficiency. Many women (and a number of physicians) feel that progesterone provides significant relief of symptoms, particularly the emotional symptoms.

It is useful for many women because of its anti-anxiety and sedative effects. This was corroborated in an early research study that was reported in the *Journal of Assisted Reproduction and Genetics*. This study found that the use of 200 mg of progesterone vaginal suppositories used twice daily for 7 months effectively reduced PMS- related symptoms.

As mentioned earlier, 80 to 90 percent of women with premenstrual tension note significant mood swings, irritability, and anxiety. These can occur for a few days to as much as several weeks out of the month. As far back as the 1930s, these mood swings were thought to be due to hormonal imbalance — specifically, estrogen excess in the face of relative progesterone deficiency.

Katharina Dalton, an English gynecologist, began treating women with progesterone thirty years ago. While this is still considered a controversial treatment, the therapeutic use of progesterone does provide relief for many women. Many of my own patients who used progesterone felt that it was tremendously beneficial and provided relief for a variety of PMS-related mood symptoms.

Progesterone is currently available over-the-counter as a topical cream, sublingual drops, rectal and vaginal suppositories or by prescription as an oral tablet.

Antianxiety and Antidepressant Medication

Both tranquilizers and antidepressants are prescribed by many physicians to treat the emotional symptoms of PMS. Benzodiazepine tranquilizers are used to calm the moods, as well as reduce anxiety and nervous tension in susceptible women. Examples of these drugs include Tranxene (chlorazapate) and Valium (diazepam). These drugs all decrease anxiety by depressing the central nervous system. They all have sedative properties, too, depending on the dose level used, and certain tranquilizers like Valium also reduce muscle tension and spasm.

Another class of mood altering drugs is the selective serotonin reuptake inhibitors (SSRIs). These medications work by blocking a receptor in the brain that reabsorbs serotonin. This helps to change the balance of serotonin, thereby helping brain cells send and receive chemical messages. The end result is an improvement in mood and behavior in women with PMS-related depression and depression in general. Commonly prescribed SSRI's include Prozac (fluoxetine), Celexa (citalopram), Zoloft (sertraline) and Paxil (paroxetine).

The main drawback with these medications is that they are slow to be effective. To begin to feel symptom relief may take between two to eight weeks, so you may not feel better when you initially begin to take these medications. It is important, however, to keep taking them since they are likely to be beneficial once their therapeutic effects start to manifest.

Women who have been taking these medications for a period of time may find that they develop withdrawal symptoms if these medications are abruptly discontinued. They should be gradually tapered off so that the brain can readjust to lower levels of these drugs. Other side-effects include nausea, dry mouth, nervousness, agitation, headache, diarrhea, reduced sexual desire, insomnia and weight gain.

The tricyclic antidepressants can also be used to treat PMS mood symptoms, particularly anxiety coexisting with depression or depression alone. These drugs such as Elavil (amitriptylene) or Sinequan (doxepin) may relieve depression by elevating levels of neurotransmitters like serotonin and norepinephrine. These are chemicals in the brain that regulate mood, personality, sleep and appetite. Imbalances in these functions are commonly seen with PMS.

Because it takes some time to build up to a therapeutic effect once treatment is initiated, there is a dangerous period of time before the drug takes hold when the patient may remain depressed and become suicidal. However, after two to three weeks of treatment, 80 percent of depressed and anxious patients notice an elevation of mood, increased alertness, and improvement in appetite.

Side effects of these drugs are fairly common. In fact, as many as one-quarter of all patients stop therapy with these drugs because of the unpleasant side effects. Many women using antidepressants will initially complain of dry mouth, blurred vision, constipation, drowsiness, or even anxiety and agitation. These symptoms tend to fade in intensity after the first few weeks of taking the medication. Sometimes, they are minimized by initiating therapy at very low doses. Other side effects include the development of shakiness or tremors in the hands; these occur in 10 percent of patients. Numbness and tingling in the arms and legs are also reported occasionally.

BuSpar™ (buspirone hydrochloride) is another antianxiety drug that can be used for the treatment of PMS. It is a very useful anti-anxiety drug that has two definite benefits over benzodiazepines and other sedatives.

First, it does not cause excessive levels of sedation, so the potentially debilitating side effect of drowsiness is decreased. Second, it is not addictive, so women using BuSpar™ do not run the risk of becoming dependent on this drug or having to go through a potentially uncomfortable withdrawal period in order to discontinue it. As a result, some physicians favor it over traditional drugs such as Xanax™ for regular use in treating generalized anxiety. Women suffering from fear, worry, tension, and irritability may benefit from this medication. It is also useful for treating the anxiety component when anxiety and depression coexist. It is less useful, however, in treating panic attacks.

Though BuSpar™ is a relatively safe drug; it should not be used with antidepressant medication belonging to the monoamine oxidase inhibitor (MAO inhibitor) classification. Interaction of these two drugs may cause an elevation in blood pressure. Also, even though BuSpar™ has been found to be less sedating than other antianxiety drugs, a woman taking it should avoid operating an automobile until she is sure that the drug does not affect her mental and motor performance.

Nervous system side effects such as drowsiness, dizziness, nervousness, and insomnia of sufficient severity to necessitate discontinuing use of the drug were seen in 3.4 percent of 2200 women studied in a clinical trial. This trial was done during the preapproval stage of testing to gather the necessary data so that the drug could be sold in the United States. In the same clinical trial, 1.2 percent of the women tested experienced digestive disturbances such as nausea severe enough to necessitate discontinuing the drug.

Other reported side effects include chest pain, tinnitus (ringing in the ears), dream disturbances, sore throat, and nasal congestion. The good news is the side effects occur in a relatively small number of patients using the drug, however. For women who tolerate the drug well the lack of physical dependence or potential for drug abuse make it a drug of choice for the treatment of generalized anxiety

There are, however, problems with the use of any medication or hormones. For example, symptoms are controlled only as long as you're on the medication. Since PMS is a long-term problem that becomes worse with age, for many women this can mean ten to twenty-five years of taking a drug or hormone. Many women either don't want to or can't be on medication for the remainder of their menstruating years. Also a doctor's prescription and careful follow-up are necessary when using drugs.

In summary, the use of medication can be extremely useful for women with moderate to severe PMS symptoms. If you do choose to use medication, I do recommend combining it with the self-help methods discussed in this book for the most thorough and complete relief.

17

Making Your Program Work

In this book, I have shared with you a complete self-care program to help prevent and relieve your symptoms of PMS and to support your radiant health and wellness.

I usually recommend beginning any self-care program slowly while you get used to the changes in lifestyle. People often differ in their ability to adjust to major lifestyle changes. Though some of my patients like to eliminate their old, unhealthy habits as quickly as possible, many other women find such rapid changes in long-term habits too stressful. Find the pace that works for you.

Enjoy the program. I always tell my patients to regard their self-care program as an enjoyable adventure. The exercises and stress-reduction techniques should give you a sense of energy and well-being. The menus and food selections I have recommended in this book provide you with an opportunity to try delicious and healthful new recipes and meal plans.

Try the treatment options that attract you the most. You may find that certain exercise routines or stress reduction techniques feel better to you than others. If that is the case, practice the ones that bring the greatest sense of relief for your particular symptoms.

Don't set up unrealistic or overly strict expectations for yourself. You don't have to be perfect to get great results. Just follow the guidelines of the program as best you can and as your schedule permits.

Remember that healing occurs in a stepwise progression. It is never a straight line. Don't feel guilty if you miss a day of exercises. It is not a major issue if you forget to take your vitamins occasionally or don't have time to exercise on a particular day. Don't be discouraged if you can't follow the dietary recommendations on vacations, holidays, or because old food cravings become too strong. Everyone falls down at times. The successful person picks herself up and moves on. Just keep going back to your goals periodically and review the general guidelines that I've outlined for you.

Be your own best feedback system. Become sensitive to what your body needs and its messages. Your body will tell you when certain foods and/or emotional stress trigger menopause related symptoms. Remember that even moderate changes in your habits can relieve your symptoms.

Periodically review the guidelines outlined in this book and continue to adapt your lifestyle to the healthful suggestions that I have shared with you from my years of medical practice. Over time you will notice many beneficial changes.

Nutrition

Make all nutritional changes gradually. Review the lists of foods to limit and foods to emphasize periodically. Each time you review this list, pick several more foods that you are willing to eliminate or try. Review these lists as often as you choose, but try to do it on a regular basis. Every small change that you make in your diet can help.

Review the guidelines for each meal. You may want to restructure a particular meal. The sample menus that I have provided in the text can serve as models for you.

Use vitamin and herbal supplements during the premenstrual period to help round out your nutritional needs. Both are very helpful for control of your PMS.

Stress Reduction

Your stress reduction exercises will help to change your belief system about your body as well as improve your autonomic nervous system function.

When you begin your program, set aside half an hour for several consecutive days and try the stress reduction exercises described in this book that appeal to you. Find the combination that works for you and then practice it regularly.

The exercises should be done on a daily basis for at least a few minutes a day. You may find that the best times to practice them are in the morning when you wake up or at night before you go to sleep. Other useful times are during the day when you are feeling particularly frazzled or stressed.

Simply take ten minutes, close the door to your room, and relax. Deep-breathe, meditate, or use the PMS visualization or affirmations. You will find that you feel much better afterward. You may also find that you enjoy doing the stress-reduction exercises before doing your regular physical exercise.

Exercise

Moderate exercise such as walking, jogging, swimming, playing tennis, or bicycling should be done on a regular basis. Every day or every other day is best.

Specific PMS Corrective Exercises

The first week or two, set aside half an hour to an hour a day for several consecutive days and do the acupressure massage, stretches, neuro-lymphatic points, and neurovascular holding points exercises that warm up, tone, and energize the entire body. Find the ones that you enjoy the most. These should always precede any specific corrective exercises for your symptoms. Find the combination of warm-ups and exercises that works best for you.

Look at the specific exercises that will correct your symptoms in the treatment chapters. Try out the exercises for your specific symptoms. Find the ones that work best for you.

Practice them on a regular basis. Starting them a few days before your PMS begins will help to prevent the symptoms.

Workbook

Use your workbook on a regular basis. It will make the program much easier and more effective for you.

The workbook pages give you a structured format with which to evaluate your habit patterns, your symptoms, and your success. The habit evaluation section will show you which areas of your life contribute to your symptoms. Check off your symptoms during the premenstrual period and list which treatments you are doing during this period to help correct them. It is important that you give yourself this feedback in an organized and easy-to-use format.

Conclusion

I hope that you enjoy the great resources that I have shared with you in this book. They have been patient proven over the years and I have been thrilled to see so many of my PMS patients benefit from them. I hope that you benefit greatly from this material and achieve the same wonderful results that my patients and I have had.

Practice PMS relieving nutritional habits, relaxation and stress reduction techniques, moderate exercise, and any specific corrective techniques that work for you to relieve your specific symptoms. Most of all -- enjoy your life each and every day.

Love,

Dr. Susan

About Susan Richards, M.D.

Dr. Susan Richards is one of the foremost authorities in the fields of family medicine and alternative medicine. Dr. Richards has successfully treated many thousands of patients emphasizing alternative health and integrative medicine in her clinical practice. Her mission is to provide her patients with safe and effective alternative therapies to greatly enhance their health and well-being.

A graduate of Northwestern University Feinberg School of Medicine, she has served on the clinical faculty of Stanford University School of Medicine and taught in their Division of Family and Community Medicine.

Her Facebook page, Dr. Susan's Healthy Living, has over one million followers. She is also an ordained minister and her ministry receives over a million prayer requests for healing each year.

NOTES

References

Atmaca M, Selahattin K, Texcan E. Fluoxetine versus Vitex agnus castus extract in the treatment of premenstrual dysphoric disorder. Human Psychopharmacol Clin Exp.2003;18:191-5.

Berger 0, Schaffner W, Schrader E, Meier B, Brattstrom A. Efficacy of Vitex agnus castus L. extract *Ie* 440 in patients with premenstrual syndrome (PMS). Arch Gynecol Obstet. 2000; 264:150-53.

Blumenthal M, Busse WR, Goldberg A, et al. The complete German Commission E. monographs: therapeutic guide to herbal medicines. Austin TX. American Botanical Council. 1998, p1694.

Borenstein JE, et al Using the dally record of severity of problems as a screening instrument for premenstrual syndrome. Obstetncs & Gynecology. 2007;109:1068

Casper RF, et at, Treatment of premenstrual syndrome and premenstrual oysphonc disorder www.uptodatecomlhomelindex.htmlAccessed Nov 23, 2011

Chapman EH, Angelica J, Spltalny G, et al Resuhs of a study of the homoeopathic treatment of PMS *JAm fnst Homeo.* 1994:87 14-21.

Cohn CM, et a! Complications of menstruation; abnormal uterine bleeding In:

Daniele C, Thompson J, Pittler MH, Ernst E. Vitex agnus castus: a systematic review of adverse events. Drug Saf. 2005;28(4):319-32.

De Souza M, Walker A, Robinson P, Bolland K. A synergistic effect of daily supplement for 1 month of 200mg magnesium plus 50mg vitamin B6 for the relief of anxiety-related premenstrual symptoms: a randomized, double-blind, crossover study. Journal of Women's Health & Gender-Based Medicine. 2000 Mar;9(2)131-3.

DeCherney AH, et at, Current Diagnosis & Treatment Obstetrics & Gynecology. 10th ed New York, NY' The McGraw-Hill Companies, 2007

Dog TL. Premenstrual syndrome. In Rakel D. Integrative Medicine. 2nd ed Philadelphia, Pa Saunders Elsevrer, 2007
http://www.mdconsult.com/daslbocklbody/2087 *46819-2/0/1494/0.* html Accessed Nov 23,2011

Frequently asked questions Gynecologic problems FAQ057. Premenstrual syndrome. American College of Obstetricians and Gynecologists. http//www.acog.org/publicationslfaq~aq057.cfm Accessed Nov 23, 2011

http://Www.accessmedicine.com/content.aspx?ald=2388399 Accessed Nov 22, 2011.

Jlng Z, et al Chinese herbal medicine for premenstrual syndrome (review). Cochrane Database of Systematic Reviews. 2009.CD006414. http://www2.cochrane.org/reviews. Accessed Dec. 6, 2011

Johnson SR. Premenstrual syndrome, premenstrual dysphoric disorder, and beyond' A clinical primer for practitioners. Obstetrics & Gynecology 2004,104:845

Panay N. Management Of premenstrual syndrome Evidence-based guidelines Obstetrics, Gynecology and Reproductive Medicine. 2011 ;21 :221.

Proctor M, Murphy P. Herbal dietary therapies for primary and secondary dysmenorrhea (Cochrane review). The Cochrane Library, Issue 2, 2002. Oxford: update software.

Shulman LP. Gynecological management of premenstrual symptoms. Current Pain and Headache Reports 2010,14367

Walker A, De Souza M, Vickers M, Abeyasekera S, Collins M, Trinca L. Magnesium supplementation alleviates premenstrual symptoms of fluid retention. Journal of Women's Health. 1998 Nov;7(9):1157-65.

Wyatt K, Dimmock P, Jones P, Shaughn O'Brien PM. Efficacy of vitamin B-6 in the treatment of premenstrual syndrome: systemic review. BMJ. 1999; 318: 1375-81.

Yakir M. Kreitler S, Brzezinski A, et al. Effects of homeopathic treatment in women with premenstrual syndrome: a pilot study. *8r Homeopath* J 2001 ;90: 148-153

Yonkers KA. et al Premenstrual syndrome The Lancet. 2008;371 1200